AF572548

Intraoperative Use of Echocardiography

Edited by
Norbert P. de Bruijn, MD
Associate Professor
Duke Heart Center
Duke University Medical Center
Durham, NC

Fiona M. Clements, MD
Assistant Professor
Duke Heart Center
Duke University Medical Center
Durham, NC

With 16 contributors

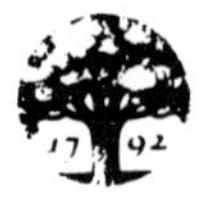

J. B. LIPPINCOTT COMPANY
Philadelphia
New York London Hagerstown

Intraoperative Use of Echocardiography

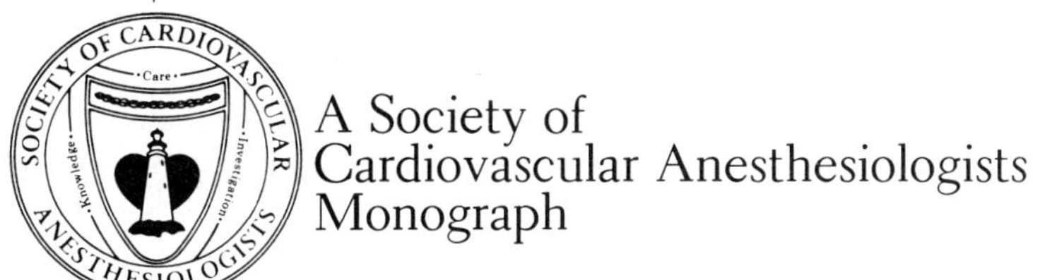

A Society of Cardiovascular Anesthesiologists Monograph

Acquisitions Editor: Nancy Mullins
Contributing Editorial Assistant: Anne Geyer
Manuscript Editor: Rosina Miller
Indexer: Nancy Weaver
Production Coordinator: Susan Clarey
Production Services: Nan Nagy
Compositor: University Graphics
Printer/Binder: R. R. Donnelley & Sons Company

1 3 5 6 4 2

Library of Congress Cataloging-in-Publication Data

Intraoperative use of echocardiography / edited by Norbert P. deBruijn, Fiona M. Clements : with 16 contributors.
p. cm.—(A Society of Cardiovascular Anesthesiologists monograph)
Includes bibliographical references and index.
ISBN 0-397-51128-0
1. Transesophageal echocardiography. 2. Heart—Surgery. 3. Intraoperative monitoring. I. De Bruijn, Norbert P. II. Clements, Fiona M. III. Series.
[DNLM: 1. Echocardiography. 2. Intraoperative Care—methods.
RD52.T73157 1991
616.1'207543—dc20
DNLM/DLC
for Library of Congress 91-6368
CIP

The authors and publisher have exerted every effort to ensure that drug selection and dosage set forth in this text are in accord with current recommendations and practice at the time of publication. However, in view of ongoing research, changes in government regulations, and the constant flow of information relating to drug therapy and drug reactions, the reader is urged to check the package insert for each drug for any change in indications and dosage and for added warnings and precautions. This is particularly important when the recommended agent is a new or infrequently employed drug.

Publication Committee of the
Society of Cardiovascular Anesthesiologists

Norig Ellison, MD, Chairman
Philadelphia, Pennsylvania

Frederick A. Burrows, MD
Toronto, Canada

Judith A. Fabian, MD
Richmond, Virginia

Simon Gelman, MD, PhD
Birmingham, Alabama

Michael Nugent, MD
Toledo, Ohio

J. G. Reves, MD
Durham, North Carolina

T. E. Stanley, MD
Durham, North Carolina

Steve Tosone, MD
Atlanta, Georgia

Margaret A. Wood, MD
Nashville, Tennessee

Contributors

Martin J. Abel, BSc, MBBCh
Assistant Professor of Anesthesiology
Mayo Medical School
The Mayo Clinic
Rochester, Minnesota

David B. Adams, RDMS
Department of Medicine, Cardiac Division
Duke University Medical Center
Durham, North Carolina

Michael K. Cahalan, MD
Associate Professor of Anesthesiology
University of California at San Francisco
School of Medicine
Director of Anesthesia for Cardiac Surgery
Moffitt/Long Hospital
San Francisco, California

Lawrence S. C. Czer, MD
Medical Director, Heart Transplant Program
Cedars-Sinai Medical Center
Assistant Professor of Medicine
University of California at Los Angeles
School of Medicine
Los Angeles, California

William J. Greeley, MD
Associate Professor of Anesthesiology and Pediatrics
Chief, Division of Pediatric Critical Care Medicine
Medical Director, Pediatric Intensive Care Unit
Duke University Medical Center
Durham, North Carolina

Zaharia Hillel, MD, PhD
Assistant Professor
Columbia University
St. Luke's\Roosevelt Hospital Center
New York, New York

Joseph A. Kisslo, MD
Professor of Medicine
Director of Echocardiography Laboratory
Duke University Medical Center
Durham, North Carolina

Jacqueline M. Leung, MD
Assistant Professor of Anesthesiology
University of California at San Francisco
School of Medicine
Veteran's Administration Medical Center
San Francisco, California

Dennis T. Mangano, PhD, MD
Professor and Vice Chairman
Department of Anesthesia
University of California at San Francisco
School of Medicine
Veteran's Affairs Medical Center
San Francisco, California

Gerald Maurer, MD
Associate Professor of Medicine
University of California at Los Angeles
School of Medicine
Director, Cardiac Non-Invasive Laboratory
Department of Cardiology
Cedars-Sinai Medical Center
Los Angeles, California

Rick A. Nishimura, MD
Associate Professor of Medicine
Department of Cardiology
Mayo Medical School
Consultant in Cardiovascular Diseases and Internal Medicine
The Mayo Clinic
Rochester, Minnesota

Nelson B. Schiller, MD, FACC
Professor of Medicine
Division of Cardiology
Director, Adult Echocardiography Laboratory
University of California at San Francisco
San Francisco, California

Khalid H. Sheikh, MD
Assistant Professor of Cardiology
Department of Medicine
Duke University Medical Center
Durham, North Carolina

Thomas E. Stanley, MD
Assistant Professor of Anesthesiology
Division of Cardiac Anesthesia
Department of Anesthesiology
Duke Heart Center
Duke University Medical Center
Durham, North Carolina

Daniel Thys, MD
Director, Department of Anesthesiology
Columbia University
St. Luke's\Roosevelt Hospital Center
New York, New York

Ross M. Ungerleider, MD
Assistant Professor of General and Thoracic Surgery
Department of Surgery
Chief, Pediatric Cardiac Surgery
Duke University Medical Center
Durham, North Carolina

Contents

Preface

Intraoperative echocardiography has gained acceptance in many operating rooms during the last decade because of its unique possibilities both as a monitor and as a diagnostic tool. Much of the development of intraoperative echocardiography has been in cardiovascular surgical procedures while the technique has been underutilized as a monitor for high-risk patients undergoing other types of surgery. The development of cheaper instrumentation should help overcome this problem.

Many problems and questions still exist about intraoperative echocardiography: Is the technique cost effective or is it just another sacrifice on the altar of the anesthesiologists' quest for more gadgets? Are anesthesiologists able to master the cognitive skills to interpret echocardiograms and if yes how could the anesthesiologists who have finished the formal part of their training attain these skills? It is our bias that the professional organizations like the SCA in close cooperation with established organizations like the American Society of Echocardiography, should play an active role in setting standards for these and other questions.

In this fifth SCA monograph we have tried to combine both clinically relevant basics of echocardiography and recent developments in the use of intraoperative ultrasound techniques. Those who are interested in pursuing this topic are advised, however, to consult some more basic texts because understanding the technical possibilities and limitations has a great impact on how effectively one can use it in everyday practice.

Norbert P. de Bruijn, MD
Fiona M. Clements, MD

Fiona Clements

1 The Evolution of the Anesthesiologist-Echocardiographer

The technique of transesophageal echocardiography (TEE) entered the sphere of anesthesiology as recently as 1985. For such alien and expensive technology to generate as much interest as it has, the results must be of real significance. Or are they? Should anesthesiologists be interested in transesophageal echocardiography, and to what extent? As this subject is still evolving, the reader will have to make up his or her own mind, and it is hoped that this volume will assist with that purpose.

Transesophageal echocardiography, like pulmonary artery catheterization, is a technique that crosses interspecialty boundaries: it has piqued the interest of cardiologists, anesthesiologists, and cardiac surgeons. Unlike pulmonary artery catheterization, however, the equipment is much more expensive, and it requires specific technical and interpretative expertise that is entirely foreign to most non-cardiologists. Anesthesiologists must now try to determine the cost-benefit ratio of TEE in our practice and must attain the necessary skill for its use. Unfortunately, cardiologists have not firmly determined the education and experience levels necessary for the qualification of *echocardiographer.* Indeed, as the technology itself has been changing so rapidly, opinions vary from institution to institution and from year to year. Some guidelines are helpful, however, and considerable cardiologic and anesthesiologic experience with TEE can be used to draw conclusions. How has this experience been gained? In what kinds of patients?

Naturally, the initial experience with TEE came from cardiologists, who were already using echocardiography for the diagnosis of heart disease, placing their ultrasound transducers on the chest wall. It was clear that imaging from the chest wall was often unsuccessful in patients with emphysema or obesity: the air in the lungs would prevent transmission of ultrasound and/or the heart would be too far from the transducer. In fact, the left atrium and ventricle, often the sites of primary interest, are also the chambers farthest from the chest wall transducer. It became obvious that a transducer positioned in the esophagus, immediately adjacent to the left chambers, could provide a good image. For the cardiologists, this development meant extraordinary success in diagnosing atrial septal defects, discovering atrial thrombi, and assessing mitral regurgitation. The left atrium and, specifically, the left atrial appendage can be searched thoroughly for thrombus. The generally higher quality images have provided more detail of cardiac anatomy, especially mitral valve and left ventricular anatomy. In addition, proximity to the descending aorta and a different perspective on the ascending aorta have increased the value of echocardiography for the diagnosis of aortic dissections.

Even with the superior quality of two-dimensional imaging, TEE would not have enjoyed the growth it has seen without the simultaneous appearance of color-flow mapping. Doppler color-flow mapping allows visualization of blood-flow velocity within the heart. This revolutionary technology has simplified the cardiac examination in many ways and made it practical to obtain detailed information about cardiac blood flow in a short space of time. The combination of Doppler color-flow mapping with a two-dimensional esophageal transducer has made intraoperative assessment of surgical repairs a feasible proposition.

Esophageal transducers are being used in a variety of locations within the hospital, such as the echo lab, the operating room, and the intensive care unit. The clinical question may be evaluated adequately with a chest wall echo; however, if images are inadequate, then almost any patient may be considered for a transesophageal examination. Some patients almost certainly need a transesophageal study. For example, patients with prosthetic mitral valves are better evaluated with esophageal images. Similarly, a good search for atrial thrombi or cardiac vegetations is better done from the esophagus. A patient who has just undergone cardiac surgery is frequently impossible to image from the chest wall. Figure 1-1 summarizes the more frequently encountered indications for TEE.

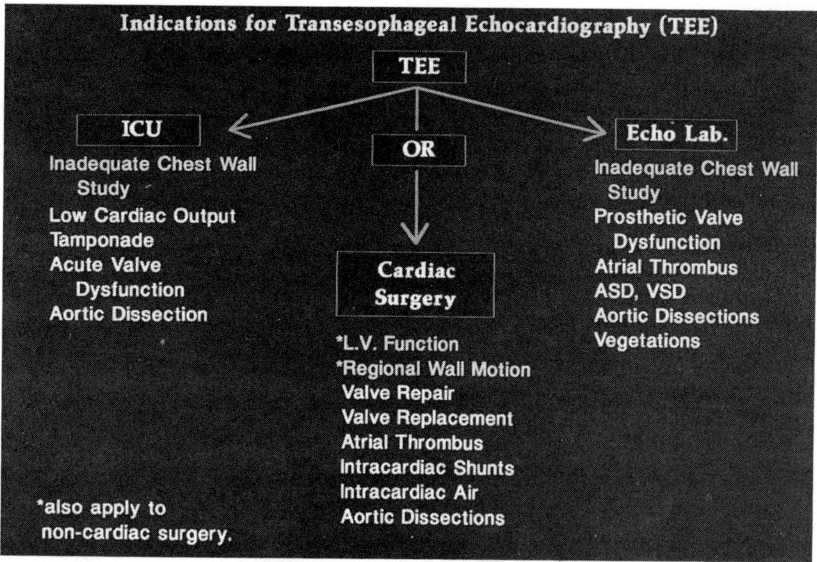

FIGURE 1-1. Indications for use of transesophageal echocardiography.

HISTORICAL BACKGROUND OF TRANSESOPHAGEAL ECHOCARDIOGRAPHY

Leon Frazin, a cardiologist, was the first to describe an esophageal transducer that he used successfully to image patients with inadequate chest wall examinations. It was capable of making only M-mode images and could not be easily controlled to select different views.[1] Directional control of the ultrasound beam was later achieved by others who housed the transducer and its wires in a fiberoptic gastroscope from which the fiberoptics were removed. This sort of assembly, which could contain a two-dimensional imaging transducer, is the forerunner of the equipment in current use. Early reports of two-dimensional transesophageal imaging came from Matsumoto and coworkers,[2,3] Hisanaga and coworkers,[4] and from Schlueter and coworkers.[5] In Europe, cardiologists were using the technique mostly in patients who were awake. Expertise was brought from Germany to the United States via Dr. Peter Kremer, who was associated with Michael Cahalan in San Francisco. Subsequently, esophageal imaging became more widely used in the United States, primarily in anesthetized patients. At the same time,

Doppler color-flow imaging had been developed in Japan and was incorporated into transesophageal imaging. This technological advance coincided with a surge of interest in repairing rather than replacing mitral valves. In addition, cardiologists had become more adventurous with balloon mitral valvuloplasty. Thus there was an instant demand for a new technology and has encouraged the use of TEE both in the echo lab in awake patients and in the operating room for evaluation of anesthetized patients.

SAFETY

By 1990, experience with TEE has accumulated; more than 10,000 uses are estimated in anesthetized patients in the United States alone and at least this number of awake studies worldwide. It is worth noting that most of the anesthetized patients have been fully heparinized for cardiopulmonary bypass. Complications have been few. Early on, Cucchiara reported a vocal cord injury felt to be caused by sustained pressure on the cord by the esophageal scope and a reinforced endotracheal tube in a patient who was undergoing a craniotomy with the neck fully flexed for several hours.[6] Curling investigated heat production at the transducer head and determined that temperatures may exceed 42°C within a few minutes at the maximum power delivery setting. However, there have been no reports of heat damage to the esophagus.[7] The largest study about safety comes from a multicenter study in Europe that involved 10,419 transesophageal uses, of which 89% were awake studies.[8] The study reported a 1.9% insertion failure rate (201 patients) due primarily to operator inexperience or patient intolerance. In 0.86% (90 patients), the study could not be completed, again primarily because of patient intolerance (65 patients). Bronchospasm, vomiting, transient arrhythmias, and angina accounted for other incomplete studies. Two patients experienced some pharyngeal or esophageal bleeding, of whom one had a malignant esophageal tumor. Whereas elective awake examinations can be accomplished with sedation and topical anesthesia in controlled conditions, concern has arisen about the risk of attempting emergency awake studies in patients with aortic dissections, for example, in whom a rise in blood pressure may be catastrophic. Matsumura and coworkers reported their experience with 72 emergency studies in awake patients, of whom 16 had acute aortic dissections.[9]

An 8% incidence of transient ischemic changes by electrocardiogram (ECG) was found, and 40% of patients had some premature atrial or ventricular beats. Patients with aortic dissections had more tachycardia and hypertension than the others. No complications were noted, however.

Overall, the safety record of TEE has been impressive. Common sense should be used: an esophageal scope should not be used in a patient with a known esophageal constriction or suspicion of esophageal varices or tumor. The plastic and rubber casing of the probe must be intact, and the electrical safety checked regularly. Low power settings should be used whenever possible, and the probe should not be moved and manipulated more than necessary.

VALUE OF TRANSESOPHAGEAL ECHOCARDIOGRAPHY: OUTCOME STUDIES

Given the effort and cost involved with the use of TEE, many are interested to know if it truly makes a difference in terms of patient management and outcome. A few investigators have tried to address these issues.

Anesthesiologists have been interested in monitoring regional left ventricular wall motion as a marker for myocardial ischemia and infarction. Two studies have reported on this topic. Smith and coworkers studied 50 patients at high risk for myocardial ischemia who were undergoing coronary or other vascular surgery and 10 normal control patients.[10] They compared the ability of TEE and ECG to detect myocardial ischemia; they also examined the relationship of intraoperative regional wall motion abnormalities and postoperative infarction. Of the high-risk patients studied, 24 out of 50 had new regional wall motion abnormalities, whereas only six had ST segment changes on the ECG. The three patients with intraoperative myocardial infarction also had persistent intraoperative regional wall motion abnormalities, but only one had ST segment changes. Persistent new regional wall motion abnormalities also occurred in three patients who did not appear to have had an intraoperative myocardial infarction. Likewise, new persistent ECG changes were noted in two patients who had no infarction. None of the ten normal patients had either regional wall motion or ST segment abnormalities.

The issue of sensitivity and specificity of the ECG or TEE is always clouded in clinical studies by the practical limitations of the techniques; in this instance, the ECG was limited to seven surface leads (including one V lead), as is standard clinical practice. It was also limited by intermittent sampling techniques, conduction abnormalities, the need for pacing, and interference from electrocautery. Transesophageal echocardiography was also limited by intermittent sampling, the observation of a single two-dimensional plane, the exclusion of much of the myocardium, and by the use of a qualitative method of regional wall motion analysis. However, given the usual clinical constraints, this study established that new persistent regional wall motion abnormalities carried a poor prognosis in terms of myocardial infarction ($p < .05$), but not every wall motion abnormality was associated with infarction. Indeed, since it is well known that the regional wall motion abnormalities produced by ischemia may not recover for hours or days after restoration of coronary perfusion, every regional wall motion abnormality need not signify simultaneous coronary ischemia or infarction.

A second study by Leung and coworkers has also examined the significance of regional wall motion abnormalities in 50 patients who were undergoing coronary artery bypass surgery.[11] The study also compared echocardiographic findings with ECG findings and hemodynamic changes. Again, regional wall motion abnormalities were seen more often than ECG changes, and postbypass TEE ischemia was related to adverse outcome in this study; as with the previous study, however, many patients with regional wall motion abnormalities did not go on to have adverse outcomes. The authors also noted that 73% of the TEE ischemic episodes occurred without demonstrable hemodynamic changes.

The available evidence, then, demonstrates that a patient without regional wall motion abnormalities almost invariably will do well; and, even though the patient with new persistent regional wall motion abnormalities has a significantly higher chance of having a perioperative myocardial infarction, most patients in this category have favorable outcomes. It is not known if therapeutic interventions can improve the outcome of those patients with regional wall motion abnormalities; however, it seems reasonable to expect that they could.

The value of transesophageal and epicardial echocardiography with Doppler color-flow mapping has also been examined in adult patients who are undergoing cardiac valve surgery. In this population, echocardiography is useful not only for prognostication but also for making intraoperative decisions regarding the surgical procedure. Sheikh and associates found that echocardiographically unsatisfactory results (i.e., valvular insufficiency or dysfunction) immediately after bypass were associated significantly with adverse outcomes.[12] Similarly, postbypass left ventricular dysfunction was associated with adverse outcome. It was also found that, in 19% of the 154 patients, a prebypass echocardiographic finding assisted or changed the planned operation. In patients with mitral regurgitation, who form the largest group of adult patients likely to benefit from intraoperative echocardiographic evaluation, Doppler color-flow mapping has been found to correlate well with angiographic evidence of mitral regurgitation.[13] In addition, it has been found that the assessment of mitral valve competence by fluid filling of the arrested left ventricle correlates poorly with Doppler color-flow mapping after mitral valve repair. Thus, TEE has now become an almost mandatory part of the mitral valve repair in many institutions. Some surgeons feel that it should be available for any valve surgery. Certainly, a good deal of reassurance is obtained from an "echo-perfect" surgical result. These results appear to apply equally to the pediatric population with congenital heart disease, in whom on-the-heart (epicardial) echo has been used intraoperatively to assess the defects and evaluate the repair.[14] The surgeon and anesthesiologist are also comforted by the ability to visualize air in the left side of the heart and document its removal. Whereas no evidence shows that the ability to visualize air or to observe left ventricular contractility specifically improves outcome, few anesthesiologists who use TEE for these purposes would doubt its usefulness.

THE FUTURE OF TRANSESOPHAGEAL ECHOCARDIOGRAPHY

Within the United States, TEE use spread rapidly during the late 1980s (Fig. 1-2). In most institutions, the cardiologists primarily appear to have taken the initiative in obtaining the equipment, with a variable degree of interest from their colleagues in anesthesiology. Few anesthesiologists have an echocardiography background and must learn the basics as they use the equipment. Many would be content with a simplified two-dimensional echo machine that would allow them to look at global left ventricular function and regional wall motion. Some effort is being devoted to this concept for intraoperative monitoring. Anesthesiologists involved with cardiac surgery, however, recognize that Doppler capability, including color-flow mapping, must be included. Some are also interested in developing a biplane system of transesophageal imaging with two orthogonal transducers situated on a single probe. This system will increase the number of available imaging planes.

Whether anesthesiologists or cardiologists should be responsible

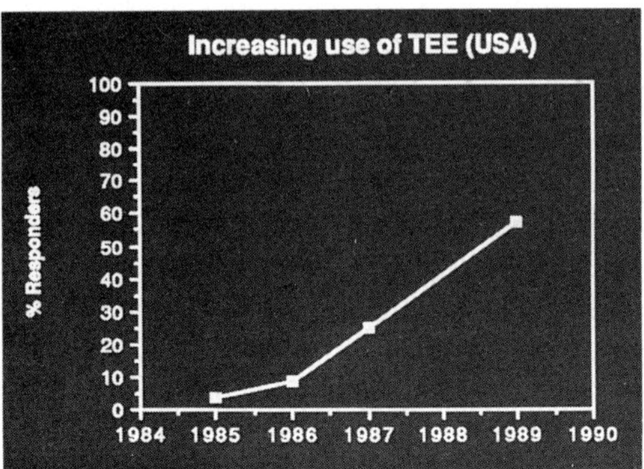

FIGURE 1-2. Increase in use of transesophageal echocardiography in recent years. Responses are from a questionnaire sent to institutions in the U.S. that have ordered or purchased TEE equipment.

for reading echo images remains a controversial issue. Since the cardiologist cannot be in the operating room continuously, it is useful for the anesthesiologist to understand cardiac imaging. A specialist in cardiac anesthesia can expect to reach and maintain a reasonable level of competence in using TEE. An on-call arrangement with a cardiologist is still an important aspect of patient care, however, when surgical decisions are to be made on the basis of echocardiographic findings.

Few cardiologists feel comfortable initially with the idea of passing a gastroscope into the esophagus of an awake patient, and fewer feel comfortable in the operating room environment. Assistance from a gastroscopist or an anesthesiologist sometimes is useful to help insert the probe. By learning to manipulate the probe and obtain different imaging planes in the anesthetized patient, the cardiologist can accelerate his or her learning curve significantly. It is also useful for the cardiologist to gain familiarity with the cardiac surgical operating room routine and environment. A patient vasodilated with isoflurane may not exhibit the same degree of mitral regurgitation as was seen preoperatively in the cardiac catheterization laboratory. Images have to be interpreted in the light of hemodynamics, the presence of cannulae in the heart, hemodilution, and other factors peculiar to the surgical situation.

Transesophageal echocardiography can be used most effectively when a good working relationship is established among the cardiologists, anesthesiologists, and surgeons. Images should be recorded on videotape and archived along with other chest wall echocardiograms, and a written report should be provided for the patient's medical record. These records can be invaluable in later follow-up of patients, especially those with valvular heart disease. At Duke University, we have a system in which the anesthesiologist records the images on videotape and dictates a report, both of which are then sent to the echo lab for review by the cardiologist. In this way, quality control is established, and the report is generated through the existing mechanism for chest wall echocardiograms.

EDUCATION FOR THE ANESTHESIOLOGIST

Formal guidelines for training anesthesiologists or others to use TEE have not been published. Certainly, it is generally felt that fellows in cardiothoracic surgery and anesthesia should be provided with some formal training, and teaching institutions that use TEE should provide such training.[15] It has been suggested that the American College of Cardiology and the American Society of Echocardiography should consider providing specific guidelines.

Guidelines entitled "Optimal Physician Training in Echocardiography" apply to chest wall echo techniques but not specifically to TEE.[16] These recommendations, however, appeared before the widespread use of Doppler color-flow imaging, which has added a new dimension to echocardiography. The recommendations of the American Society of Echocardiography include three levels of training. A Level 2 is considered adequate experience for taking independent responsibility for echocardiographic studies and includes approximately 300 two-dimensional and M-mode studies in addition to 225 Doppler examinations over approximately 6 months time, during which the physician's effort is primarily (75%) directed toward the study of echocardiography. These recommendations do provide a framework with which anesthesiologists can compare their experiences with TEE.

In most institutions that perform TEE in the operating room, we are seldom concerned with M-mode imaging. The majority of Doppler studies involve color-flow imaging rather than conventional Doppler. However, a working familiarity with conventional Doppler is certainly desirable for the more accurate description of valvular lesions. Obtaining images with TEE is easier than with conventional chest wall echocardiography because only a limited number of views can be examined; the quality of the images is also better. For these reasons, and when confined to an adult population of patients who have coronary or valvular surgery, a level of competence appropriate to the operating room setting can probably be achieved more easily than that described for the broader-based cardiologist-echocardiographer.

The "echo training program" for fellows in cardiac anesthesia at many institutions continues to evolve. At Duke University, we are fortunate to have established a close working relationship with the hospital's busy echo lab, which performs over 1000 echo studies per month. This volume provides a number of cases far in excess of the 1000 studies per year suggested as a minimum acceptable case load for a training program.[16] Our fellows spend 6 to 8 weeks assigned to the echo lab, during which time they have no primary responsibilities for patient care. They learn the basics of ultrasound technology, perform and observe chest wall studies, and attend daily reading sessions. Through interactions with the cardiology faculty and the echocardiographers, they learn to produce high-quality images through the appropriate use of the gain controls and other electronic processing. They are also responsible for attending all transesophageal studies, in and out of the operating room, as the primary operator when appropriate. During the remainder of the year-long clinical part of the fellowship, they do other transesophageal studies on their own cardiac surgical patients on a daily basis. This situation is enabled by the availability of an echo machine and two echo-scopes permanently stationed in the operating room. Regular exposure to intraoperative echocardiography, therefore, occurs over the entire year. In addition, cardiology fellows who acquire experience in TEE spend time in the cardiac operating rooms, and attending cardiologists are frequent visitors. A case load of approximately 1500 open heart operations per year ensures sufficient volume for trainees. In this situation, we feel that a cardiac anesthesia fellow achieves training analogous to a Level 2 experience appropriate to the operating room setting. The fellow is also expected to learn to interact well with cardiologists and to know when he or she needs to consult a cardiologist for an intraoperative interpretation, knowledge that is perhaps one of the most important facets of training.

Echocardiography has undergone great developments during the past 10 years. We can expect further changes and refinements to take place, and continuing education will be a major challenge if we are to keep pace with the technology. Echocardiography seems to have become firmly planted within the sphere of cardiac anesthesia and surgery. It seems reasonable to expect that noncardiac anesthesia will involve echocardiography if and when less expensive and simpler equipment becomes available. Our responsibility, therefore, is to concern ourselves with the education of residents in this technology and make known to the manufacturers what equipment anesthesiologists need.

References

1. Frazin L, Talano JV, Stephanides L et al: Esophageal echocardiography. Circulation 54:102, 1976
2. Matsumoto M, Oka Y, Strom J et al: Application of transesophageal echocardiography to continuous intraoperative monitoring of left ventricular performance. Am J Cardiol 46:95, 1980
3. Matsumoto M, Hanrath P, Kremer P et al: Evaluation of left ventricular performance during supine bicycle exercise by transoesophageal M-mode echocardiography in normal subjects. Br Heart J 48:61, 1982
4. Hisanaga K, Hisanaga A, Nagata K, Ichie Y: Transesophageal cross-sectional echocardiography. Am Heart J 100:605, 1980
5. Schleuter M, Langenstein BA, Polster J et al: Transoesophageal cross-sectional echocardiography with a phased array transducer system: Technique and initial clinical results. Br Heart J 48:67, 1982
6. Cucchiara RF, Nugent M, Seward JB et al: Air embolism in upright neurosurgical patients: Detection and localisation by two-dimensional transesophageal echocardiography. Anesthesiology 60:353, 1984
7. Curling PE, Newsome LR, Rogers A et al: 2D-transesophageal echocardiography: A bidirectional phased array probe with temperature monitoring (abstr). Anesthesiology 61:120, 1984
8. Daniel WG, Angermann C, Curtius J et al: Practicability and safety of transesophageal echocardiography: A European multicenter study (abstr). Circulation (suppl) 80:340, 1989
9. Matsumura M, Shah P, Kyo S et al: Electrocardiographic and hemodynamic changes during emergent transesophageal examination in cardiovascular diseases. Circulation (suppl) 80:340, 1989
10. Smith JS, Cahalan MK, Benefiel DJ et al: Intraoperative detection of myocardial ischemia in high-risk patients: Electrocardiography versus two-dimensional transesophageal echocardiography. Circulation 72:1015, 1985
11. Leung JM, O'Kelly B, Browner WS et al: Prognostic importance of postbypass regional wall motion abnormalities in patients undergoing coronary artery bypass graft surgery. Anesthesiology 71:16, 1989
12. Sheikh KH, de Bruijn NP, Rankin JS et al: The utility of transesophageal echocardiography and Doppler color flow imaging in patients undergoing cardiac valve surgery. J Am Coll Cardiol 15:363, 1990
13. Czer LS, Maurer G, Bolger AF et al: Intraoperative evaluation of mitral regurgitation by Doppler color flow mapping. Circulation (suppl) 76:108, 1987
14. Ungerleider RM, Greeley WJ, Sheikh KH et al: The use of intraoperative echo with Doppler color flow imaging to predict outcome after repair of congenital cardiac defects. Ann Surg 210:526, 1989

15. Goldman ME, Mindich BP, Nanda NC: Intraoperative echocardiography: Who monitors the flood once the flood gates are opened? J Am Coll Cardiol 11:1362, 1988
16. Pearlman AS, Gardin JM, Martin RP et al: Guidelines for optimal physician training in echocardiography: Recommendations of the American Society of Echocardiography Committee for Physician Training in Echocardiography. Am J Cardiol 60:158, 1987

Daniel M. Thys
Zaharia Hillel

2 How It Works: Basic Concepts in Echocardiography

PROPERTIES OF ULTRASOUND

Echocardiography is the procedure that uses *ultrasound* (sound above human audible range) to probe the heart and great vessels. The ultrasound is sent into the thoracic cavity and is partially reflected by the cardiac structures. From these reflections, information on distance, velocity, and density of objects within the chest is derived.[1]

Basic Concepts: Wavelength, Frequency, Velocity

An ultrasound beam is a continuous or intermittent train of waves emitted by a *transducer* (wave generator). The beam is composed of density or pressure waves and can exist in any medium with the exception of vacuum (Fig. 2-1). Ultrasound waves are characterized by their wavelength, frequency, and velocity. *Wavelength* is the distance between the two nearest points of equal pressure or density in an ultrasound beam; *velocity* is the speed at which the waves propagate through a medium. At any fixed point in the path of a beam of ultrasound waves that are traveling through a medium, pressure waves are set up; these waves oscillate regularly and continuously between high and low values. The number of cycles (oscillations) per second is called the *frequency* of the

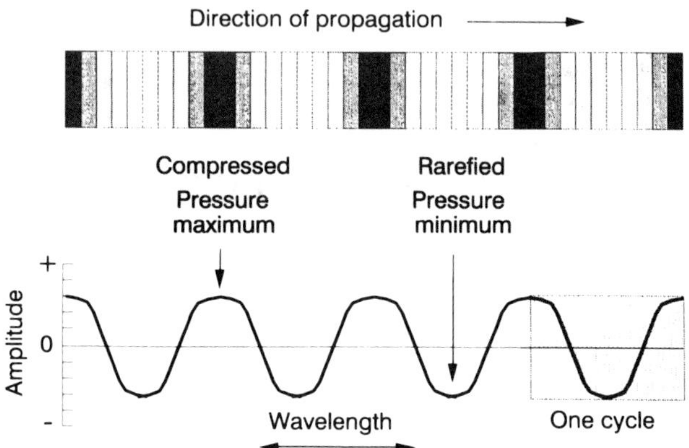

FIGURE 2-1. A sound wave is a series of compressions and rarefactions. The combination of one compression and one rarefaction represents one cycle. The distance between the onset (peak compression) of one cycle to the next is the wavelength.

wave. Ultrasound frequencies are always higher than 20,000 cycles per second (hertz or Hz), which is the upper limit of the human audible range. The relationship between the frequency (f), wavelength (λ), and velocity (v) of a sound wave is defined by Equation 2-1.

$$v = f \cdot \lambda \tag{2-1}$$

The velocity of sound varies with the properties of the medium through which it travels. For soft tissues, this velocity approximates 1540 m/s. Because the frequency of an ultrasound beam is determined by the properties of the emitting transducer, while the velocity is a function of the tissues through which the sound travels, wavelengths must vary to maintain the relationship shown in Equation 2-1.

Propagation: Attenuation, Reflection, Scatter

Waves interact with the medium in which they travel and with one another. Interaction among waves is called *interference.* The manner in which waves interact with a medium is determined by its density and homogeneity. When a wave is propagating through an inhomogeneous

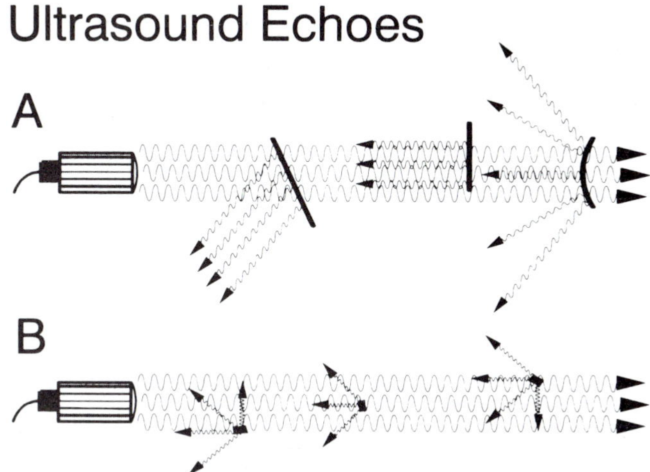

FIGURE 2-2. *A*, Specular echoes originate from relatively large, strongly reflective, regularly shaped objects with smooth surfaces and are relatively intense and angle dependent. *B*, Scattered echoes originate from small, weakly reflective, irregularly shaped objects and are less angle dependent and less intense.

medium, and all living tissues are essentially inhomogeneous, it is partly absorbed, partly reflected, and partly scattered (Fig. 2-2). Reflected echoes, also called *specular echoes*, are usually much stronger than scattered echoes. A grossly inhomogeneous medium, such as a stone in a water bucket or a cardiac valve in a blood-filled heart chamber, produces strong specular reflections at the water-stone or blood-valve interface. Conversely, media that are inhomogeneous at the microscopic level, such as muscle, produce more scatter than specular reflection. Specular reflections are obtained when the width of the reflecting object is larger than one fourth of the wavelength of the ultrasound. It follows that in order to visualize smaller objects, ultrasound of shorter wavelength must be used. Since the velocity of sound in soft tissue is approximately constant (1540 m/s), shorter wavelengths are obtained by increasing the frequency of the ultrasound beam (Equation 2-1). Although more useful in visualizing small objects, higher frequencies compared to lower frequencies produce more scatter when meeting tissue inhomogeneities and, thus, generate more confusing signals.

Any ultrasound beam that travels through tissues is weakened or attenuated as it progresses. Table 2-1 gives the distance in various tissues at which the intensity or amplitude of an ultrasound wave of

TABLE 2-1. Half-Power Distances for Tissues and Substances Important in Echocardiography

Material	Half-Power Distance (cm)
Water	380
Blood	15
Soft Tissue (except muscle)	5–1
Muscle	1–0.6
Bone	0.7–0.2
Air	0.08
Lung	0.05

2 MHz is halved (the half-power distance). Clearly, echo studies across lung or other gas-containing tissues are not feasible. Nor are they feasible across dense structures, such as bone, or strongly scattering tissues, such as thick muscle.

Modern ultrasound transducers employ piezoelectric crystals to transmit ultrasound and receive echoes. A high frequency electronic signal causes the crystal to vibrate and emit ultrasound of the same frequency. Conversely, reflected ultrasound echoes that strike the crystal's surface generate vibrations, which the crystal converts to electronic signals. These signals when amplified and processed can be imaged on a television screen. Electronic circuits measure the time delay between the transmitted and received signals. Using the known speed of ultrasound in tissue, the time delay is converted into a precise distance measurement from transducer to tissue.

Commonly used transducers spend a small amount of time, typically about 1 microsecond (10^{-6} seconds), to emit a pulse of ultrasound waves. They then "listen" for the returning echoes for about 0.25 millisecond and pause for 0.75 millisecond or less before repeating the cycle. Ultrasound takes about 0.1 millisecond to travel through 10 cm of human tissue and to be reflected or echoed back to the transducer. Time is not lost in the reflection process itself.

IMAGING TECHNIQUES

M-Mode

The most basic form of ultrasound imaging is *M-mode* echocardiography. In this mode, the density and position of all tissues in the path of a narrow ultrasound beam, that is, along a single line, are displayed as

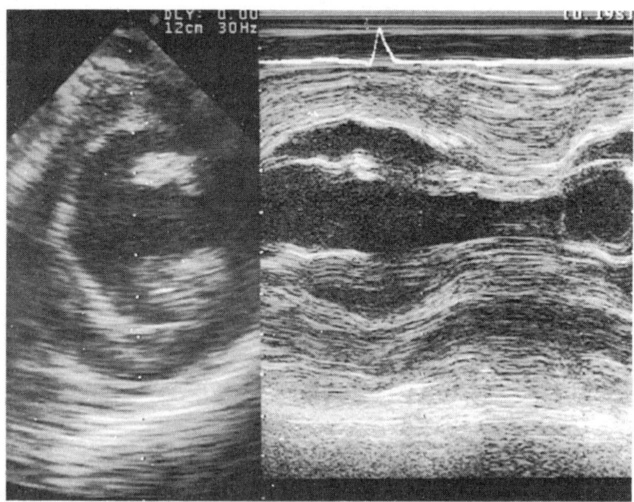

FIGURE 2-3. Split-screen display of the left ventricular short axis at the level of the papillary muscles. *Left,* Two-dimensional image with the M-mode cursor *(white dots)* positioned in the center of the cavity. *Right,* Time display of the M-mode signal. Time is on the horizontal axis while the cardiac structures are displayed along the vertical axis. The systolic inward motion of the endocardium can be visualized.

a scroll on a video screen. The scrolling produces an updated, continuously changing time plot of the studied tissue section, several seconds in duration (Fig. 2-3). Since this is a timed *motion display* (normal cardiac tissue is always in motion), it is called M-mode. Since only a limited part of the heart is being observed at any one time and because interpretation of the image requires considerable skill, M-mode is not currently used as a primary imaging technique. This mode, however, is useful for the precise timing of events within the cardiac cycle and is often used in combination with color-flow Doppler for the timing of abnormal flows (see below). Quantitative measurements of size, distance, and velocity are also easily performed in the M-mode without the need for sophisticated analysis equipment. Whenever a measurement includes a temporal component, the M-mode image is more advantageous than a two-dimensional image because it is updated 1000 times each second. Thus, more subtle changes in motion or dimension can be appreciated.

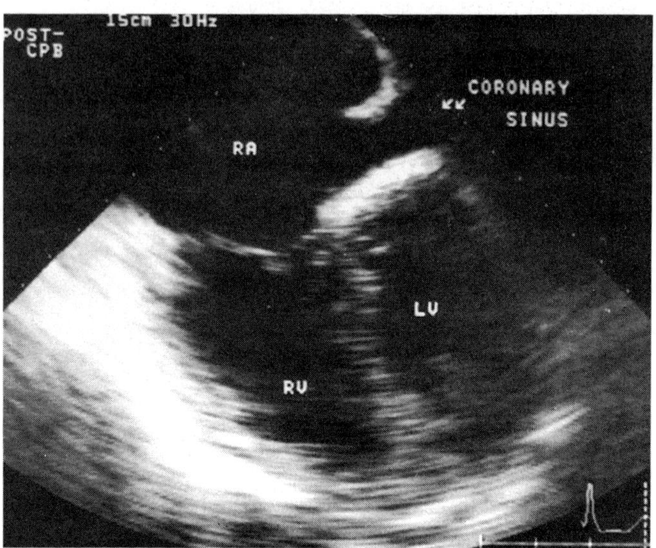

FIGURE 2-4. Two-dimensional basal view of the heart at the level of the coronary sinus. This image demonstrates that the two-dimensional mode is well suited for the visualization of anatomic structures. ***RA***, right atrium; ***RV***, right ventricle; ***LV***, left ventricle.

Two-Dimensional Mode

By rapid, repetitive scanning along many different radii within an area in the shape of a fan (sector), echocardiography generates a two-dimensional image of a section of the heart. This image, which resembles an anatomic section and thus can be more easily interpreted, is called a *two-dimensional scan* (Fig. 2-4). Information on structures and motion in the plane of a two-dimensional scan is updated 30 to 60 times per second. This produces a "live" (real-time) image of the heart. Two-dimensional echo devices scan the heart by using either a mechanically steered transducer or, as is common in many of the newer devices, an electronically steered ultrasound beam (phased-array transducer).

DOPPLER TECHNIQUES

The Doppler Effect

Information on blood-flow dynamics can be obtained by applying Doppler frequency shift analysis to echoes reflected by the moving red blood cells.[2,3] Blood-flow velocity, direction, and acceleration can be instantaneously determined. This information is different from that obtained in two-dimensional imaging and, hence, complements it.

The Doppler principle as applied in echocardiography states that the frequency of ultrasound reflected by a moving target (red blood cells) is different than the frequency of the emitted ultrasound. The magnitude and direction of the frequency shift are related to the velocity and direction of the moving target. The velocity of the target is calculated with the Doppler equation

$$v = \frac{cf_d}{2f_o \cos \theta} \tag{2-2}$$

in which v is the flow velocity, c the velocity of sound in tissue (1540 m/s), f_d the frequency shift, f_o the frequency of the emitted ultrasound, and θ the angle between the ultrasound beam and the direction of blood flow (Equation 2-2).

The only ambiguity in Equation 2-2 is that, theoretically, the direction of the ultrasonic signal could refer either to the emitted or the received beam. By convention, however, Doppler displays are made with reference to the received beam, and, thus, if the blood flow and the reflected beam travel in the same direction, the incidence angle is 0° and the cosine is +1. As a result, the frequency of the reflected signal is higher than the frequency of the emitted signal.

Equipment used in clinical practice shows blood-flow velocities as waveforms. The waveforms consist of a display of the spectral analysis of velocities on the ordinate with time on the abscissa (Fig. 2-5). On such a display, blood flow toward the transducer is by convention represented above the baseline. If the blood flows away from the transducer, the incidence angle is 180°, the cosine equals −1, and the waveform is displayed below the baseline. When the blood flow is perpendicular to the ultrasonic beam, the incidence angle is 90° or 270°. The cosine of either angle is 0 and no frequency shift is detected. The inclusion of the cosine of the incidence angle in the Doppler equation results in the observation that blood-flow velocities are measured most accurately when the ultrasonic beam is, as nearly as possible, parallel (or antiparallel) to the direction of blood flow. In clinical practice, deviations from parallel up to 20° can be tolerated, since they contribute an error of 6% or less.

Most modern echo scanners combine Doppler capabilities with two-dimensional imaging capabilities. After the desired view of the heart has been obtained by a two-dimensional scan, the Doppler beam, represented by a cursor, is superimposed on the two-dimensional image. The operator positions the cursor as parallel as possible to the

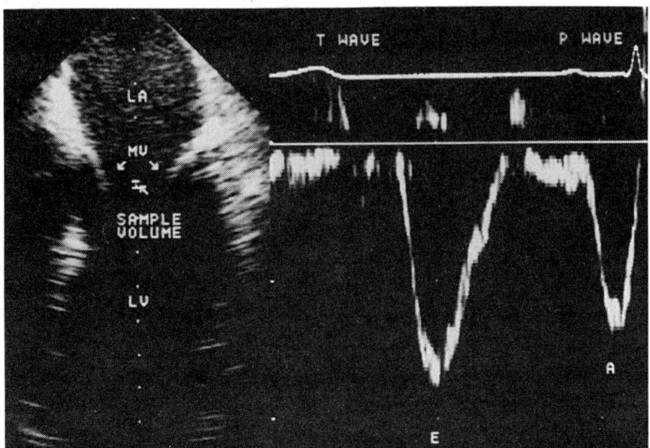

FIGURE 2-5. Split screen image with two-dimensional and pulsed-wave Doppler images. *Left,* Basal view of the heart. *LA,* left atrium; *LV,* left ventricle; *MV,* mitral valve. The sample volume indicates the location of the Doppler velocity sampling. *Right,* Spectral display of the Doppler velocity signals over time. Time is on the horizontal axis while velocity is on the vertical axis. The early ventricular filling peak *(E)* occurs after the T wave on ECG, and the atrial filling peak *(A)* follows the P wave. The velocity signals are displayed below the baseline because flow is away from the transducer.

assumed direction of blood flow and then empirically adjusts the direction of the beam to optimize the audio and visual representations of the reflected Doppler signal. At present, Doppler technology can be used in at least four different ways to measure blood velocities: these are pulsed-wave, high–pulse-repetition frequency, continuous-wave, and color-flow Doppler. Although each of these methods has specific applications, they are seldom concurrently available and then only on the most sophisticated and expensive echocardiographic devices.

Pulsed-Wave Doppler

In pulsed-wave Doppler, blood-flow parameters can be determined at precise locations within the heart by emitting repetitive short bursts of ultrasound at a specific frequency (pulse-repetition frequency or PRF) and analyzing the frequency shift of the reflected echoes at an identical sampling frequency (f_s). A time delay between emission of the ultrasound signal burst and sampling of the reflected signal determines the depth at which the velocities are sampled. The delay is proportional to the distance between the transducer and the location of the velocity measurements. To sample at a given depth (D), sufficient time must be allowed for the signal to travel a distance of $2 \cdot D$ (from the transducer to the sample volume and back). The time delay, T_d, between the emission of the signal and the reception of the reflected signal is related to D and to the speed of sound in tissues (c) by the formula in Equation 2-3.

$$D = \frac{c \cdot T_d}{2} \qquad (2\text{-}3)$$

The operator varies the depth of sampling by varying the time delay between the emission of the ultrasonic signal and the sampling of the reflected wave. In practice, the sampling location or *sample volume* is represented by a small marker on the monitor screen. It can be positioned at any point along the Doppler beam by moving it up or down the Doppler cursor. On most devices, it is also possible to vary the width and height of the sample volume.

The trade-off for the ability to measure flow at precise locations is that ambiguous velocity information is obtained when flow velocity is high. A simple reference to Western movies clearly illustrates this point (Fig. 2-6). When a stagecoach gets underway, its wheel spokes are observed as rotating in the correct direction. As soon as a certain speed is attained, however, rotation in the reverse direction is noted. This reversal occurs because the camera frame rate is too slow to correctly observe the motion of the wheel spokes. In pulsed-wave Doppler, the ambiguity exists because the measured frequency shift (f_d) and the sampling frequency (f_s) are in the same frequency range (kHz). Ambiguity is avoided only if the Doppler frequency shift is less than half the sampling frequency (Equation 2-4).

$$f_d < \frac{f_s}{2} \qquad (2\text{-}4)$$

The expression $f_s/2$ is also known as the Nyquist limit. Doppler shifts above the Nyquist limit create artifacts described as *aliasing* or *wrap-around,* and blood-flow velocities appear in a direction opposite to the conventional one (Fig. 2-7). Blood flowing with high velocity toward the transducer results in a display of velocities above and below the

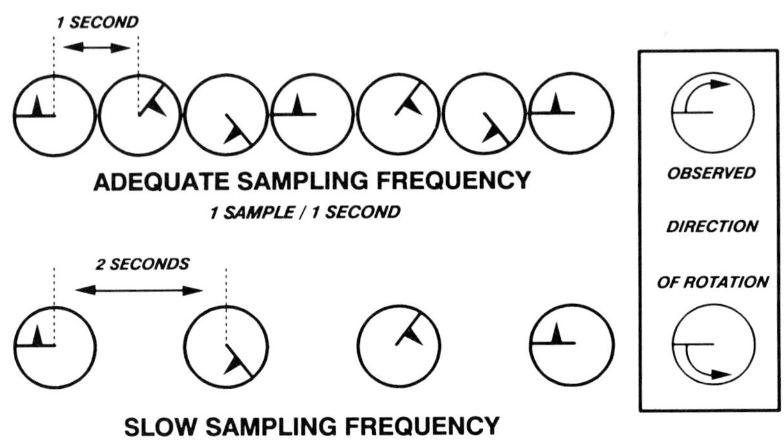

FIGURE 2-6. Diagram illustrates the importance of sampling frequency. If a wheel rotates clockwise at a speed of 1 rotation every 3 seconds, a sampling frequency of 1 sample every second results in correct display of the direction of rotation. With a sampling frequency of 1 sample every 2 seconds, the observed direction of rotation is reversed.

baseline. This artifact can be avoided by increasing the sampling frequency. This action, in turn, limits the time available for a pulse to travel to the sample volume and back, thus limiting the range. The relationship between the maximal detectable velocity and the range at which it can be detected is known as the range-velocity product or V_mR,

$$V_mR = \frac{c^2}{8f_o} \qquad (2\text{-}5)$$

in which V_m is the maximal velocity that can be unambiguously measured and R is the range or distance from the transducer at which the measurement is to be made (Fig. 2-8, Equation 2-5). Pulsed-wave Doppler measurements are performed with the transducers used for two-dimensional imaging.

High–Pulse-Repetition Frequency Doppler

On some instruments, pulsed-wave Doppler can be modified to a high–pulse-repetition frequency (high-PRF) mode. While in conventional pulsed-wave Doppler only a single burst of ultrasound is considered to

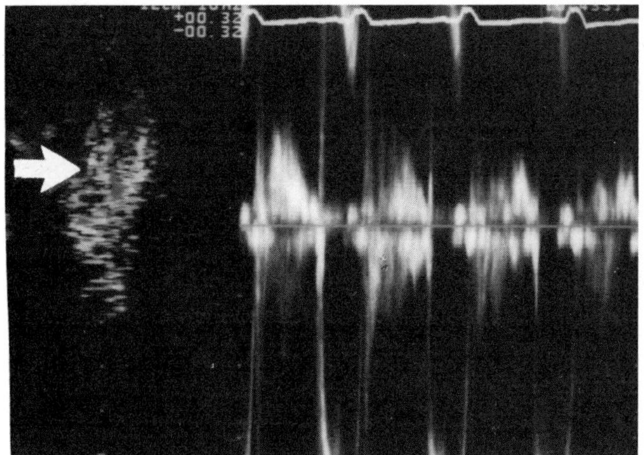

FIGURE 2-7. Aliasing in pulsed-wave Doppler sampling. *Left,* Basal two-dimensional view of the heart at the level of the mitral valve. The location of the sample volume is indicated by the *arrow. Right,* The peak velocity of blood flow across the mitral valve exceeds the Nyquist limit (± 0.93 m/s), and the highest flow velocities away from the transducer are displayed above the baseline *(top of the panel).*

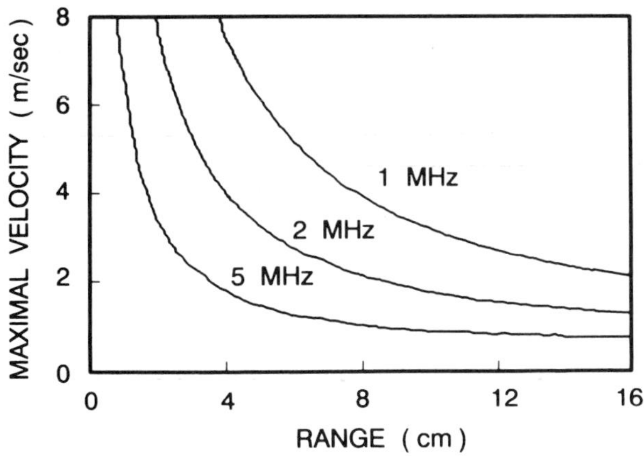

FIGURE 2-8. The range-velocity product.

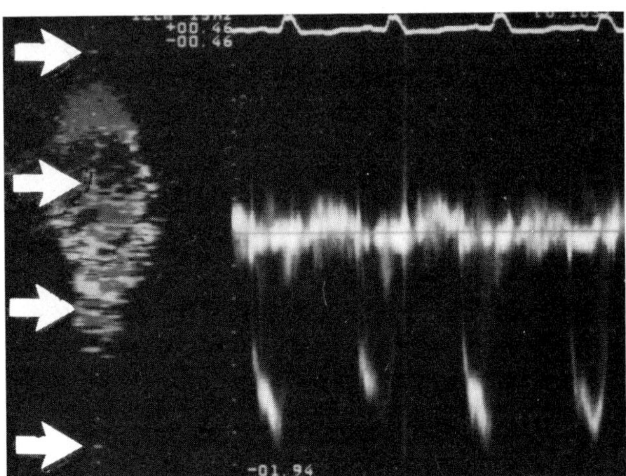

FIGURE 2-9. High–pulse repetition sampling of blood-flow velocity at the level of the mitral valve in the same patient as in *Figure 2-7.* With high-PRF, the Nyquist limit is raised to $\pm$ 1.94 cm^{-1}, and aliasing is eliminated.

be in the body at any given time, in high-PRF Doppler, two to five sample volumes are simultaneously present in the tissues. Information coming back to the transducer may be coming back from depths of either two, three, or four times the initial sample volume depth (range gate). The returning signals can be a mix of signals that have been emitted early and have traveled to distant gates and signals that were sent late and returned from the first-range gate.

The high-PRF mode allows the sampling frequency to increase since the scanner does not wait for the return of the information from distant gates (Fig. 2-9). Nonetheless, it receives that information back within the specified time-gate period. Higher velocities can be measured with this method than with pulsed-wave Doppler; however, the depth from which the velocity signals are reflected is unknown (range ambiguity).

Continuous-Wave

The continuous-wave Doppler technique uses continuous, rather than discrete, pulses of ultrasound waves. As a result, the region in which flow dynamics are measured can not be localized precisely. Blood-flow velocity is, however, measured with great accuracy even at high flows.

While many echo scanners have both pulsed-wave and continuous-wave Doppler capabilities, most transesophageal probes, used for two-dimensional imaging, cannot perform continuous-wave measurements. Dedicated continuous-wave probes have two transducers, one of which continuously emits ultrasound while the other continuously receives echoes.

Continuous-wave Doppler is particularly useful for the evaluation of patients with valvular lesions or congenital heart disease. These patients typically exhibit high-velocity intracardiac blood flows. Continuous-wave Doppler is also the preferred technique with which to attempt to derive hemodynamic information from Doppler signals.

Color-Flow Mapping

Recent advances in electronics and computer technology have made possible color-flow Doppler ultrasound scanners. They display blood flow within the heart in colors and in real time, while also imaging the tissues by two-dimensional technique. The images produced by these devices show the location, direction, and velocity of cardiac blood flow,

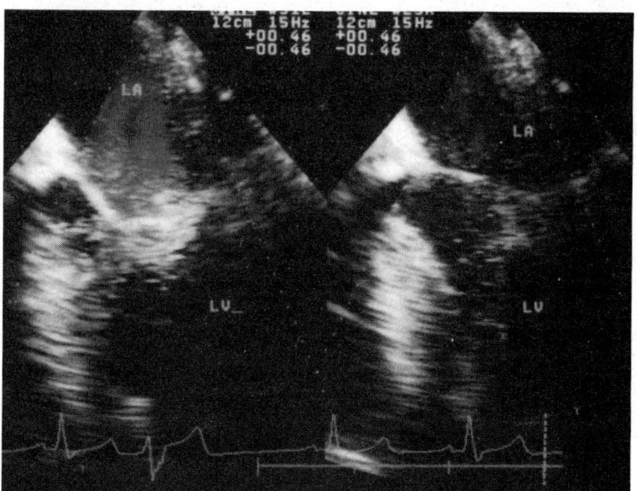

FIGURE 2-10. Diastolic and systolic color-flow Doppler images of the left heart. *LA,* left atrium; *LV,* left ventricle. *Left,* Diastolic flow is away from the transducer and displayed in blue. *Right,* Systolic flow is toward the transducer and displayed in red.

and allow one to estimate flow acceleration and distinguish between laminar and turbulent blood flow. An example of a color-flow Doppler image is shown in Figure 2-10. Color-flow Doppler echocardiography is based on the principle of multigated, pulsed-wave Doppler.[4] According to this principle, blood-flow velocity is sampled at many locations, along many lines, covering the entire imaging sector. At the same time, the sector is also scanned to generate a two-dimensional image of the tissues.

Doppler color-flow imaging uses the three basic colors (red, blue, and green) used in a standard color television. Each picture element (pixel) on the video monitor screen displays a particular combination of the colors. Where the scanner detects blood flow in a direction toward the transducer (the top of the image sector), the color red is shown. At locations where flow away from the transducer is detected, the color blue is displayed. This color assignment is completely arbitrary and is determined by the equipment's manufacturer. In the most common color-flow coding scheme, more rapid blood-flow velocity (up to a limit) is exhibited as more intense color. The color green is added to either red or blue when flow velocities change by more than a preset value within a brief time interval (exhibit flow "variance"). Both rapidly accelerating

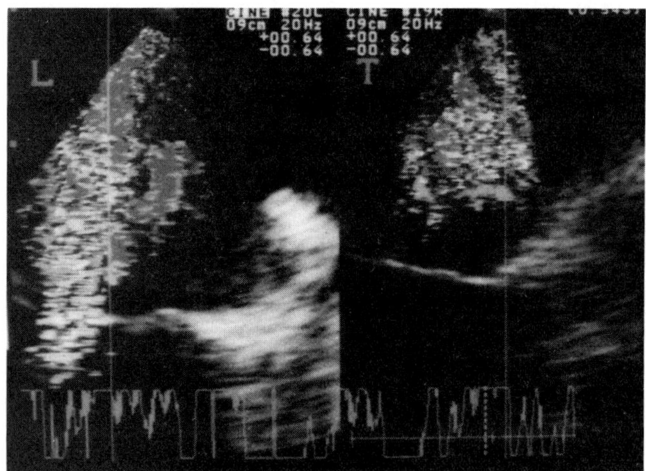

FIGURE 2-11. Color-flow Doppler images at the level of the mitral valve in a patient with severe mitral regurgitation. Longitudinal *(L)* and transverse *(T)* representations of the regurgitant jet were obtained with the use of a biplane transesophageal transducer. The mosaic pattern and multiple colors are typical for regurgitant lesions.

laminar flow (change in flow speed), as well as turbulent flow (change in flow direction) satisfy the criteria for rapid changes in velocity and, therefore, are mapped in colors with added green. With the addition of green to red or blue, a whole range of intermediate colors, including yellow, cyan, magenta, and white, can be displayed. In areas where highly turbulent flows are detected, such as in regurgitant jets, a mosaic of all the above colors is often noted. An example of this type of color-coding map is demonstrated in Figure 2-11.

EQUIPMENT

Ultrasound Scanners

The conversion of reflected ultrasound echoes into two-dimensional images is a complicated process that involves numerous electronic and digital manipulations.

Basic Principles

A two-dimensional echo image is generated by scanning the heart every 17 ms, or 60 times each second. The image generated from a single .0166-second scan is called a *field. Interlacing* combines two scans or fields into a frame of .0333-second duration. Since the human brain cannot interpret an image that lasts only .0333 second, a microprocessor can further modify the frame electronically, before it is displayed, while still operating in real time. The intrinsic persistence of the television screen enhances image quality, and the end result is a fairly smooth picture when a continuous sequence of frames is displayed.

Resolution

Resolution is the ability of ultrasound to distinguish fine detail. The resolution of an echo system is the minimum distance that must separate two distinct reflectors so that they can be imaged as separate entities. Image resolution is markedly different along the two major image axes. The axial resolution of a pulsed instrument (resolution along the direction of the beam) is approximated in Equation 2-6.

$$\text{Axial Resolution} = \frac{0.77 \times \text{Number of Cycles per Pulse}}{\text{Transducer Frequency}} \qquad (2\text{-}6)$$

The typical acoustic transducer resolution for a 5 MHz transducer with a narrow, three-cycle pulse duration is calculated in Equation 2-7.

$$\frac{0.77 \cdot 3}{5} \approx \underline{0.5\text{mm}} \tag{2-7}$$

Lateral resolution is the minimum distance, perpendicular to the ultrasound beam, at which two distinct objects can be imaged as separate. It is determined almost entirely by the beam diameter; the narrower the beam, the higher the lateral resolution. Typical values for lateral resolution are 2 to 3 mm. Axial resolution is better than lateral resolution because, along the axis of the beam, tissue information is imaged as it is detected; in the lateral direction, the image is formed by the juxtaposition of many different line scans.

Preprocessing

Ultrasound echoes are received and converted to analog electronic signals by the transducer. In most modern echo scanners, these signals undergo several modifications before being digitized, further manipulated, and eventually displayed as an image. Preprocessing describes those modifications performed on analog or digital signals before input into the scanner's digital memory. These include dynamic-range manipulation, gain attenuation, time-gain compensation, and leading-edge enhancement.

Dynamic-Range Manipulation. The intensity of echo signals spans a wide range from weak to strong. Strong signals that fall beyond the saturation level of the electronic circuitry and weak signals that fall below the sensitivity of the instrument are cut off. The dynamic range (DR) of an ultrasound scanner is defined by these cut-off limits and can be adjusted by the operator (Fig. 2-12). In this manner, signals of low intensity that contain little useful information, but mostly noise, can be selectively rejected.

A wide DR is needed for high resolution, while a narrow range facilitates discrimination between true image signals and unwanted noise. In clinical echocardiography, both strong signals that arise from dense tissues, such as cardiac valves, and weaker signals that arise from soft tissues, such as myocardium, are of interest. To give the weaker signals greater representation in the DR, an amplifier converts the linear signal-intensity scale into a logarithmic scale. While this conversion increases the sensitivity of detection for weaker signals, it also, unfortunately, tends to amplify noise.

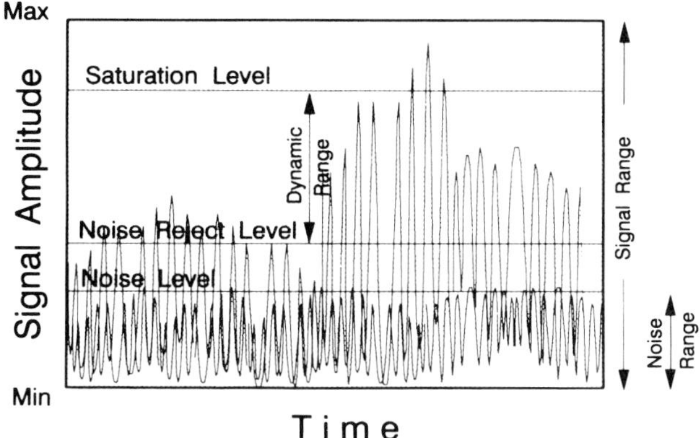

FIGURE 2-12. This diagram represents the dynamic range of a representative echocardiographic display system. All ultrasound signals begin at zero signal level and can increase in amplitude until they reach the signal "saturation" level. Many of the low-intensity signals fall within the range of the background noise and are, therefore, obscured. All systems have a built-in system reject, which eliminates both the system noise and the low-intensity echoes that lie just above the noise level. The dynamic range of the system is between the noise reject level and the saturation level. Signals within the dynamic range appear on the image display.

Gain, Attenuation, and Damping. The gain and attenuation controls of a scanner increase or decrease the intensity of all signals in a proportional manner. As a result, they change the number of detected echo signals by bringing them above or below the rejection threshold of the dynamic range. To deal with the potential loss of image quality caused by the display of the larger number of insignificant echoes obtained at high gain settings, a "damping" adjustment exists. Damping does not modify the received signal directly, but it decreases the strength of the emitted ultrasound beam by limiting the duration of the pulses that form the beam. Since less power is sent toward the target, fewer noise echoes are generated. Damping also enhances the image since it improves resolution by decreasing the number of cycles in each ultrasound pulse (see Equation 2-6).

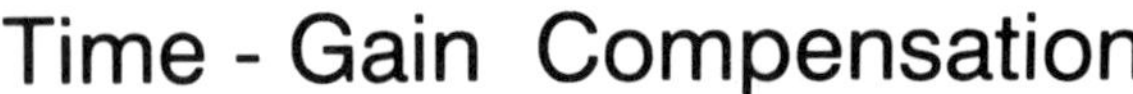

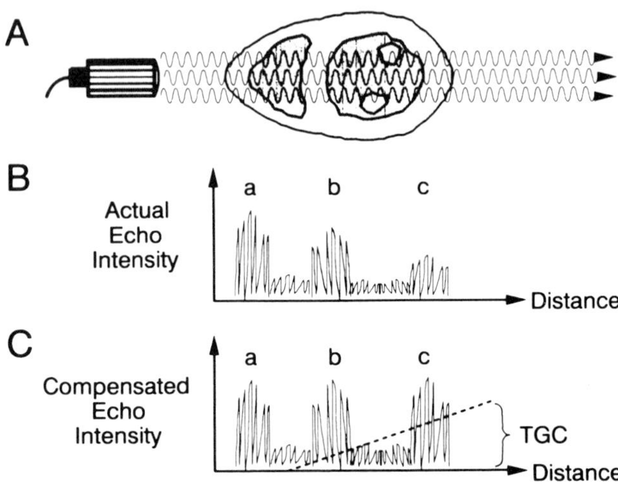

FIGURE 2-13. *A,* As an ultrasound beam is aimed across the heart, specular echoes are reflected at the right ventricular wall *(a),* the septum *(b),* and the left ventricular wall *(c). B,* The normal loss in echo strength is due to the decreasing intensity of the beam as it propagates through the heart. *C,* Time-gain compensation (TGC) allows the intensity of the far-field signals to be increased selectively.

Time-Gain Compensation. Since any wave that travels through tissues is attenuated to a degree proportional to the traveled distance, it is necessary to compensate for the fact that echoes that return from more distant objects are weaker than those from equally dense objects closer to the transducer. A mechanism called *depth compensation,* or *time-gain compensation,* is used to achieve this compensation. The manner in which time-gain compensation is implemented is illustrated in Figure 2-13. It can be controlled manually or automatically.

Leading-Edge Enhancement. Leading-edge enhancement, or differentiation, is another type of preprocessing used to sharpen the video image. The reflected echo signal undergoes half-wave rectification and is smoothed into a signal envelope (Fig. 2-14A, B). An amplifier then differentiates the leading edge of the smoothed signal envelope to its first mathematical derivative (Fig. 2-14C), and a narrower

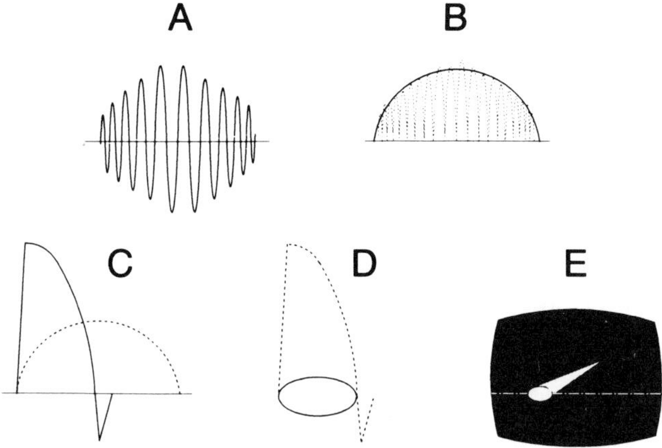

FIGURE 2-14. Leading-edge enhancement techniques. *A*, Radiofrequency (RF) type of echo display. *B*, This video display represents the average height of the upper half of the RF signal. *C*, Differentiation is obtained by taking the first derivative of the video display. *D*, Intensity modulation represents the conversion of signal amplitude to intensity, changing the signal from a spike to a dot. *E*, Display of the signal on the video screen.

and brighter image spot is formed (Fig. 2-14D). Since a two-dimensional echo image is composed of multiple radially juxtaposed scan lines, excessive edge enhancement narrows bright spots in the direction of the travel of the echo beam, that is, axially but not laterally. For this reason, leading-edge enhancement is primarily performed on M-mode scans, while instruments with two-dimensional capability use little or no edge enhancement in that mode. Therefore, M-mode images often have better resolution than two-dimensional images and are better suited for quantitative measurements.

Postprocessing

Digital Scan Conversion. After analog preprocessing is completed, ultrasound devices digitize the image data with an analog-to-digital (A-D) converter (Fig. 2-15). Further processing is done while data are stored in the digital memory (input processing) or as they are read from the memory (output processing). An early step in digital processing uses a scan converter to transform the information obtained as

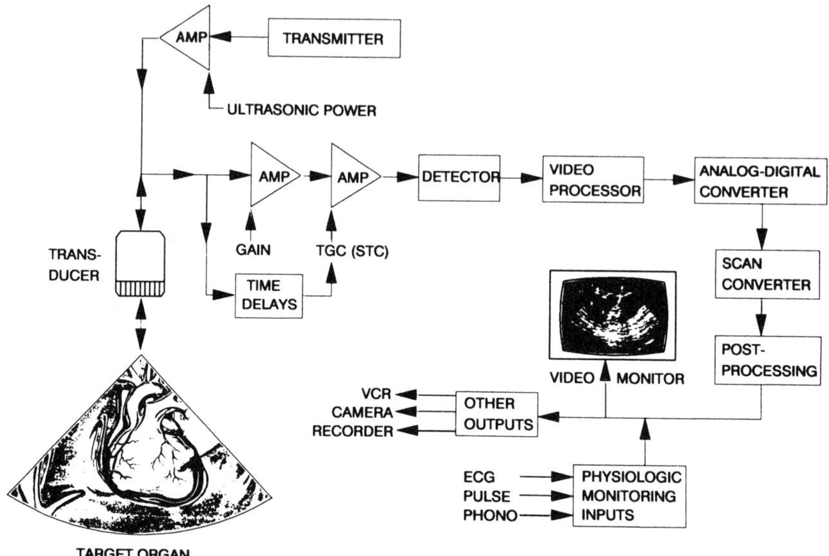

FIGURE 2-15. Schematic of a modern ultrasound scanner. The *arrows* indicate the directions for the flow of information or electronic power. *AMP*, electronic amplifier; *TGC (STC)*, time-gain compensation; *VCR*, video cassette recorder.

radial sector scan lines into a rectangular (Cartesian) format for television screen display.

The memory stores the information of two adjacent scan fields that consist of a total of 128 scan lines. Each scan line is assigned to one column of memory. One row of memory is also assigned for each of the 512 horizontal television image lines (raster lines). Therefore, a typical television display of an echo image consists of 128 columns by 512 rows for a total of 65,536 picture elements or pixels. While the monitor only displays 64 shades of gray for each pixel, the memory unit assigned to each pixel has the capacity to store 1024 degrees of brightness. Each pixel is assigned 10 binary bits of memory for a total of 2^{10} (1024) possible different values.

Temporal Processing. As digital data are entered into memory, they can undergo temporal averaging in one or two modes. In the variable-persistence mode, information from previous images is combined with current image data. A weighted average of the old and new data is then entered in memory as the new current data. A built-in mechanism allows variable representation of old data into the new image. A different input-processing option calculates the arithmetic mean of the new data and up to nine frames of existing data.

Input processing is mainly used to improve the signal-to-noise ratio. In a two-dimensional echo image, a lower signal-to-noise ratio translates into a less granular image appearance (the result of microscopic scatter) and less echo dropout (the result of weak signals that are difficult to detect on the screen). Time averaging is most useful to enhancing slowly varying images.

Histogram Equalization. The video image is generated from data retrieved from memory via the scan converter. During retrieval, data can be subjected to histogram equalization. This process redistributes the original gray level assignment of each pixel according to the relative frequency of occurrence of the particular gray level in the entire image, in equal fashion. All levels of gray receive some representation, even though the original image may have been formed from a narrower range of gray levels.

Gray-Scale Processing. Each unit of memory assigned to a pixel can store 1024 values of echo intensity, while the pixel itself can only display 64 shades of gray; thus, each gray level represents multiple echo intensities. The gray level is reassigned by transfer functions of variable shapes, slopes, and end points. An inverting transfer function allows the M-mode display to exist as a dark background with white lines or as a light background with dark lines. Gray-scale processing greatly affects image quality.

Spatial Processing or Convolution Operations. Spatial processing is a sophisticated type of averaging that involves modifications in the content of a pixel based on the content of its neighbors. In Figure 2-16A, the gray level at pixel A_{25} is replaced by the average gray level of all pixels within the "kernel" W_1 through W_9, or, simply stated, by the average of itself and the eight surrounding gray levels ($A_{25} = .1111 [A_{14} + A_{15} + A_{16} + A_{24} + A_{25} + A_{26} + A_{34} + A_{35} + A_{36}]$). This operation is done for all pixels, and the new pixels are stored in a new image memory area. This process produces spatial smoothing of the image and is particularly useful for parts of the image in which no abrupt changes in the echo density occur. It also eliminates noise. When the detection of subtle changes in density is desired, such as in endocardial border detection, or edge enhancement, a different convolution process is used. Applying the kernels shown in Figure 2-16B, the new A_{25} value

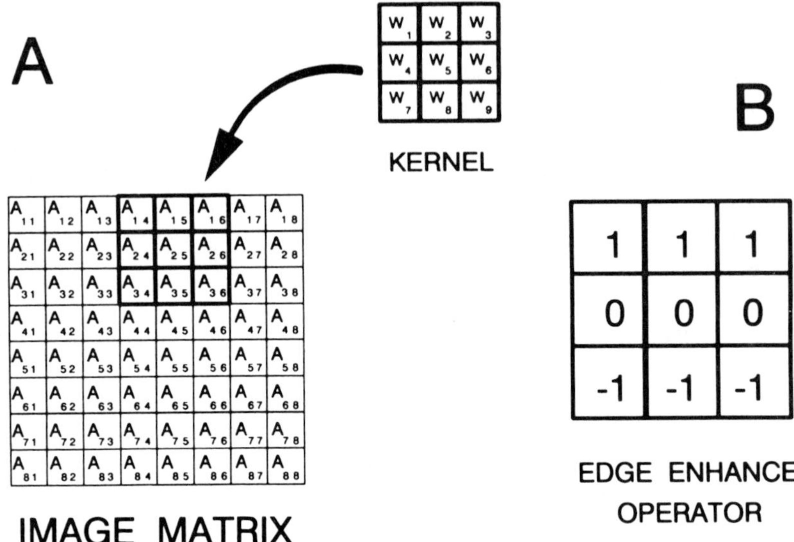

FIGURE 2-16. Digital-spatial processing by convolution operators.

would be $A_{25} = .1111\ (A_{14} + A_{15} + A_{16} - A_{34} - A_{35} - A_{36})$. To enhance vertical edges, a similar transformation can be used with the values of the kernel mask rotated 90°. Edge enhancement has limited success because most ultrasound image edges are relatively smooth, and the enhancement operator works best with images in which light and dark regions change abruptly.

Manufacturers

Several ultrasound companies manufacture echo scanners that accommodate transesophageal transducers. These companies include the following:

Acuson (Mountain View, CA)
Aloka-Corometrics (Wallingford, CT)
ATL (Bothell, WA)
Ausonics (Milwaukee, WI)
Diasonics (Milpitas, CA)
GE Medical Systems (Milwaukee, WI)
Hewlett-Packard (Andover, MA)
Hoffrel (South Norwalk, CT)
Kontron (Everett, MA)

Siemens (Iselin, NJ)
Toshiba (Tustin, CA)
Vingmed/Interspec (Philadelphia, PA)

While scanners share many common features, they do differ significantly in important, as well as trivial, details. For specific details on any particular device, the reader is referred to the particular manufacturer's technical manuals. Most scanners are of a size comparable to a medium refrigerator and contain the following components:

1. Scanner electronics (hidden from view)
2. Control panel(s)
3. Transducer port(s) (connectors)
4. Viewing video monitor(s)
5. Video cassette recorder (optional, but invariably included: VHS, Beta, or Super-VHS format)
6. Photography unit (optional, usually a Polaroid unit)
7. Hard copy display (paper chart recorder, optional)
8. Speaker(s) for generating sound of the same frequency as the Doppler shift (happens to be in the audible range)
9. Additional monitoring channels: ECG, pressure (optional), sound (optional)

Transducers

In echocardiography, the goal is to aim ultrasound waves at a given tissue section and subsequently to receive undistorted echoes from that tissue section alone. Different transducers accomplish this task with varying efficiency. The simplest device uses a single, small piezoelectric element, which produces a wide beam of circular, concentric ultrasound waves. The problem with this simple system is that it generates echoes indiscriminately from tissues in all directions around it; hence, it has poor resolution and does not locate objects well.

A more advanced transducer consists of a linear array of crystals that emit synchronously. Each individual crystal produces its own circular ultrasound waves. The end result is a planar (flat) beam that moves in a direction perpendicular to the array. For some distance away from the transducer, the width of this beam is approximately the same as the width of the array, a fact which allows the beam to interrogate tissues selectively. A single large-element transducer can produce the same effect.

Even the straightest parallel beam, however, eventually diverges after it has traveled a certain distance from the transducer. This distance (L), or depth of field, at which the beam is no longer parallel is estimated as a formula

$$L = \frac{D^2}{\lambda} \tag{2-8}$$

in which D represents the size of the transducer surface (Equation 2-8). The depth of field sets the limit for the practical depth of the ultrasound examination. From Equation 2-8, it appears that the larger the transducer, or the smaller the ultrasound wavelength, the greater the depth of field. To generate two-dimensional echo images, the transducer must be able to scan the target field with a linear arc or sector scanner. In clinical echocardiography, either mechanical or electronic (phased-array) two-dimensional sector scanners are used.

Mechanical

In mechanical transducers, an oscillating or rotating transducer head is used to scan the tissues. M-mode and two-dimensional examinations can be performed but only in a sequential manner. Since the scanning is performed by rotation of the transducer head, the electronic analysis device or echoscanner can be relatively small.

Phased-Array

Electronic scanners use linear phased-array transducers, which can contain as many as 128 piezoelectric elements. Electronic beam steering is achieved by multiple circuits, each of which provides a properly delayed electric impulse to their dedicated array element. Wave summation produces a planar or flat wave front at any desired angle within a theoretical 180° sector (Fig. 2-17). In practice, however, scanning transducers are limited to sectors of approximately 90°. A significant advantage of the electronic phased-array scanner is that it can simultaneously display two-dimensional as well as M-mode images. In a phased-array scanner, the returning echoes are received selectively. Using similar time delays as in ultrasound emission, a phased-array scanner can "focus" the reception of signals from specific tissue locations.

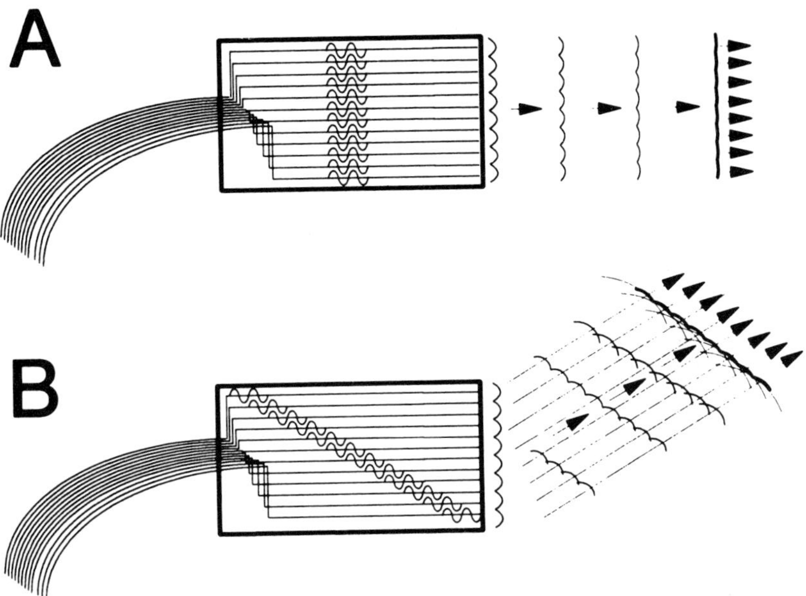

FIGURE 2-17. Method of beam transmission and steering in the phased-array format. *A*, A series of electrical pulses is depicted moving from left to right toward the transducer elements in the array. The pulses activate the elements, simultaneously producing a series of small wavelets. As these wavelets move away from the transducer face, they summate to form a beam that propagates away from the transducer. *B*, The transducer elements are activated slightly out of phase. In this example, the lower transducer is activated first, producing an acoustic wavelet that propagates away from the array. Rapidly thereafter, the other elements are activated in sequence, each producing a wavelet slightly behind the preceding one. The individual wave fronts are summated to produce an acoustic beam that approximates in shape and direction the beam that would be produced by a transducer aimed in that direction.

Annular Phased-Array

Annular (circular) phased-array technology has been recently paired with a mechanical scanner in a transesophageal probe (Vingmed/Interspec, Philadelphia, PA). In an annular array, the piezoelectric elements are ring shaped; hence, the ultrasonic beam has circular symmetry. This property allows the beam to be focused within the specific scan plane, as well as along each of the individual lines of the two-dimensional sector. Because image scanning is mechanical, simultaneous two-dimensional and pulsed-wave Doppler or M-mode imaging are impeded. However, continuous-wave Doppler velocity measurements are possible with this type of probe (one ring serves as the transmitter while another serves as the receiving crystal).

Transesophageal

Single-Plane Transducer

The standard transesophageal transducer for intraoperative use is based on the flexible gastroscope concept (Fig. 2-18). Most adult-size probes are approximately 100 cm long and 9 to 12 mm in diameter. The width at the transducer tip is often a couple of millimeters larger than the shaft diameter. The probes have either three or four degrees of motion. Two of these are linear motion (sliding) along the esophagus and rotation along the length of the shaft. In addition, all probes have greater than or equal to 90° up-down (flexion-extension, third degree of freedom) and most newer probes have less than or equal to 90° left-right motion at the tip. The last two types of motion are controlled by knobs at the proximal end. Due to the distensibility of the esophagus and lack of rigidity of the surrounding anatomic structures, the orientation of the tip does not always correspond to the control settings. The

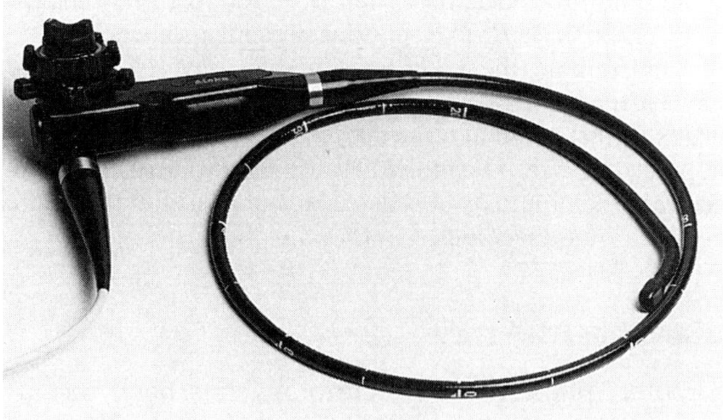

FIGURE 2-18. A modern transesophageal transducer *(Aloka-Corometrics, Wallingford, CT)* with bidirectional motion of the tip. It interfaces with a standard echoscanner and has M-mode and two-dimensional imaging, as well as pulsed-wave, high-PRF, and color-flow Doppler capabilities.

probe tends to rotate along its length while the transducer tip is being oriented. For most transesophageal echocardiography probes, phased-array technology is used.

Multiplane Transducer

BIPLANE. A biplane transesophageal probe (Aloka-Corometrics, Wallingford, CT) has been introduced recently. This probe has two similar phased-array transducers mounted side by side. One transducer scans in a direction perpendicular to the probe shaft (transverse scanning), while the other scans longitudinally (parallel to the shaft). The probe is 100 cm long and 13.5 mm in diameter, while the distance between the center points of the two transducers is 1 cm. Each has 32 elements and operates at a frequency of 5 MHz. With this probe, transverse and longitudinal scanning can be performed in alternating fashion, but not simultaneously. Due to the finite separation between the two elements, slight repositioning of the probe may be necessary to image precisely the same segment of tissue with the longitudinal and transverse transducers. The perceived advantages of the biplane probe are that a large number of new tomographic cuts can be obtained with the longitudinal transducer and that intracardiac jets can be visualized in orthogonal planes.

MATRIX. A new technical development in probes circumvents the problem of center-point separation in biplane imaging. Omoto and colleagues have recently introduced a new transesophageal probe with a matrix phased-array biplane transducer.[5] This transducer allows true orthogonal scanning of the heart without repositioning of the probe or switching between two elements. A single two-dimensional array of crystals can be phased to alternately scan along as well as perpendicularly to the axis of the probe by mere use of a switch. This probe interfaces to a standard commercial scanner. No readily identifiable differences in image quality could be detected between the matrix and the standard biplane probes in patients.

PEDIATRIC. Recently, smaller esophageal transducers have been introduced for pediatric flexible gastroscope examinations.[6] One such probe (Aloka-Corometrics, Wallingford, CT) has a 5 MHz transducer with 26 elements. The transducer's dimensions are 14 mm by 6.4 mm by 6.8 mm, and it is mounted on a 70-cm flexible gastroscope (Fig. 2-19). This probe has been used to image congenital cardiac malformations not visualized by standard transthoracic exam.[7] It also allows

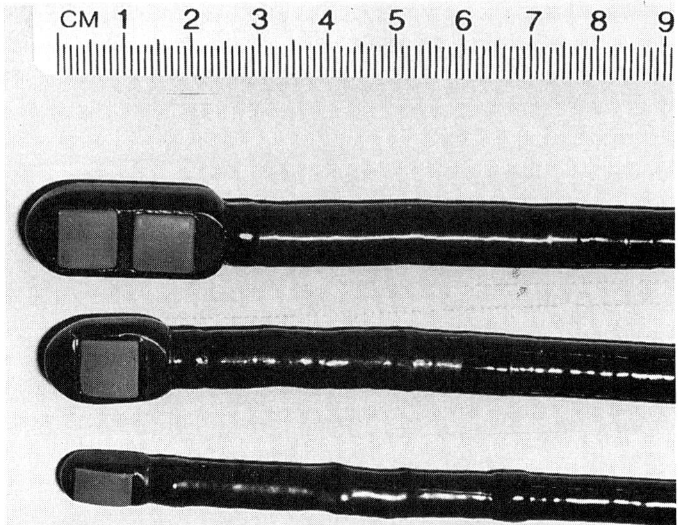

FIGURE 2-19. Transducer heads for the biplane *(top)*, standard *(middle)*, and pediatric *(bottom)* transesophageal probes (*Aloka-Corometrics, Wallingford, CT*).

intraoperative and continuous assessment of cardiac function and surgical interventions in newborns and small infants.

THREE DIMENSIONAL. More recently, an experimental probe has been introduced which allows three-dimensional imaging of cardiac anatomy by reconstruction from multiple, precision, planar-scan images.[8] A computer-driven micromanipulator controls the scan planes, and a computer integrates the final images. Single-plane imaging was performed with a standard phased-array scanner. In this fashion, left ventricular volumes and ejection fraction were measured in dog hearts. Excellent agreement was obtained between the three-dimensional reconstructed transesophageal ultrasound data and corresponding radionuclide and thermodilution measurements.

Image Analysis Methods and Devices

On nearly all the ultrasound devices, the operator has the ability to manually "freeze" or store a single image frame on the screen. This allows visualization and close scrutiny of any unusual transient anatomic or physiologic observation. It also allows one to perform quantitative measurements on line. Using this storage mode, however, it is somewhat difficult to capture a particular point in the cardiac cycle. For this reason, modes that acquire more than a single frame have been devised.

Cine Memory

One of the more modern modes of information storage is cine memory. When activated, this mode captures in digital memory approximately 1 second's worth of high-fidelity image information. The information can then be played back in several different ways. It can be replayed frame by frame, using a manually controlled track ball to step between frames. This feature allows the observer to spend any amount of time on any one frame. It can also be replayed continuously in repeating, endless-loop fashion, either at the same speed at which it was recorded or at a slower speed, allowing scrutiny of brief transient observations.

Videotape

The video recorder is the most common long-term, mass-storage medium used in echocardiography. All devices come with or can be equipped with a 1/2″ VHS videocassette recorder (VCR) very similar to the VCR for home use. Higher resolution "Super-VHS" or professional (3/4″) VCRs are also available. Since the VCR is an analog type of storage medium, the quality of videotaped images is currently inferior to the real-time display or the digital cine-memory replay. This fact makes quantitative and sometimes qualitative image analysis more difficult.

Other Storage Media (Paper Chart, Photography, Digital Storage)

Photographic or digital paper chart recorders are available for most devices and are most useful for off-line, quantitative measurements of M-mode data scrolled in time (continuous time record). These devices can also provide prints of single frame two-dimensional images. Prints of color-flow Doppler images are obtained using either an instant Polaroid-type camera or a regular 35 mm camera with color film.

In addition to the standard photographic color record, high-fidelity color prints can be produced with color video printers (Mitsubishi, Piscataway, NJ, and others) from any digital or video source.

Digital image storage is possible on magnetic disk. Standard floppy disks can store only a limited number of images since the amount of information in a single full video frame is about 1 megabyte (MB) or 10^6 bytes. Furthermore, current hardware and computer architecture do not allow rapid retrieval of image information. A new digital mass storage medium uses "write-once/read-many" digitally encoded laser disks. Using a large 810 MB memory, it can store 24,000 frames or 800 different cine loops each 30 frames long.

Quantitative Image Analysis

On-Line Analysis. All new echo devices and most of the older systems have built-in, computer-driven quantitative image-analysis packages. Analysis can be performed either on an individually stored "frozen" frame or on any frame played back from cine memory. For M-mode data, lengths, velocities, and time intervals can be measured.

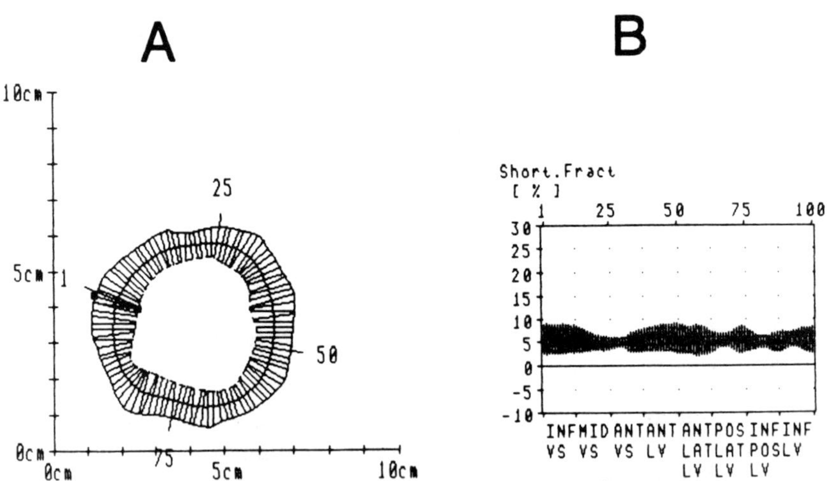

FIGURE 2-20. Off-line analysis of left ventricular wall motion. *A,* The inward motion of the endocardium during systole was measured by the device along 100 chords perpendicular to the center line between the end-systolic and end-diastolic endocardial outline. *B,* The systolic motion *(solid line)* is compared with the standard deviation of the motion measured in normal subjects *(vertical lines).*

For two-dimensional or color-flow images, lengths, areas, and angle relations can be measured. This information can then be substituted into formulas to obtain anatomic-physiologic parameters, such as wall thickness, wall motion, cavity diameter, the area or volume of a cardiac chamber, and area or volume ejection fraction. From Doppler data, velocity, acceleration, stroke volume and cardiac output (needs two-dimensional information also) are measurable. All these measurements require some operator input in the form of pointing or line tracing on the video screen using a track ball or joystick. Doppler power spectra can be traced automatically once their beginning and end are identified. Automatic border tracing (endocardium or epicardium) of two-dimensional images has just been introduced and will soon appear in commercial scanners (Hewlett-Packard, Andover, MA).

Off-Line Analysis. Off-line image analysis can be performed on video data. The data can be acquired from the scanner, in digital format, by a special data analysis station, or from videotape playback on such a device. With direct digital retrieval, image quality is high, but only limited amounts of information can be stored. The videotape stores tens of thousands of images but of a lower quality. All the on-line analysis features are available on off-line analysis stations. In addition, more sophisticated operations, such as wall-motion or wall-thickening analysis with digital readout and graphing as a function of image position, are possible (Fig. 2-20).

References

1. Thys DM, Hillel Z, Konstadt SN, Goldman ME: Intraoperative Echocardiography. In Kaplan JA (ed): Cardiac Anesthesia, 2nd edition. Orlando, Grune & Stratton, 1987
2. Hatle L, Angelsen B: Doppler Ultrasound in Cardiology, 2nd edition. Philadelphia, Lea & Febiger, 1984
3. Kisslo J, Adams D, Mark DB: Basic Doppler Echocardiography. New York, Churchill Livingstone, 1986
4. Kisslo J, Adams DB, Belkin RN: Doppler Color Flow Imaging. New York, Churchill Livingstone, 1988
5. Omoto R, Kyo S, Matsumura M et al: Biplane color Doppler transesophageal echocardiography: Its impact on cardiovascular surgery and further technological progress in the probe, a matrix phased-array biplane probe. Echocardiography 6:423, 1989
6. Ritter SB, Thys DM: Pediatric transesophageal color flow imaging: Smaller probes for smaller hearts. Echocardiography 6:431, 1989
7. Ritter S, Hillel Z, Narang J et al: Transesophageal real time Doppler flow

imaging in congenital heart disease: Experience with a new pediatric transducer probe. Dynamic Cardiovasc Imag 2:92, 1989
8. Martin R, Graham M, Kao R et al: Measurement of left ventricular ejection fraction and volumes with three-dimensional reconstructed transesophageal ultrasound scans: Comparison to radionuclide and thermal dilution measurements. J Cardiothoracic Anes 3:260, 1989

Michael K. Cahalan

3 Detection of Intraoperative Myocardial Ischemia with Two-Dimensional Transesophageal Echocardiography

Within seconds after interruption of myocardial blood flow, normal inward motion and thickening of the affected myocardium ceases. No other pathophysiologic process produces such acute changes in segmental myocardial contraction. Until recently, anesthesiologists could not detect these changes because they had no way of directly monitoring myocardial contraction. Fortunately, the situation changed with the advent of two-dimensional transesophageal echocardiography (TEE). This chapter reviews studies pertinent for the use of TEE as an intraoperative monitor for myocardial ischemia.

STUDIES IN ANIMALS

In 1935, Tennant and Wiggers observed that acute coronary ligation resulted in paradoxical motion in the ischemic area.[1] Many subsequent studies further refined the observation. For instance, Forrester and colleagues demonstrated that in the presence of a severe coronary constriction, segmental contraction decreased linearly as a function of segmental coronary blood flow: hypokinesia progressed to dyskinesia as coronary perfusion pressure fell from 100 to 20 mm Hg.[2] Subsequently, segmental contraction abnormalities or wall motion abnormalities (SWMA) have been shown to occur within seconds of the onset of regional ischemia[3] and simultaneously with regional lactate production.[4]

Battler and colleagues compared segmental myocardial contraction and ST segment change during ischemia.[5] They induced graded reductions in coronary blood flow in a canine model. Segmental myocardial contraction was measured with implanted sonomicrometers and the electrocardiogram (ECG) recorded from intracardiac and body-surface leads. During mild partial occlusion of a coronary artery, segmental myocardial contraction decreased 17%, intracardiac derived ST segments elevated significantly, but no change occurred in the body surface ECG for the 10 minutes of partial occlusion. With more severe coronary constriction, systolic wall thickening further decreased, and both surface and intracardiac ECGs showed significant ST changes. However, ST changes appeared 1 to 5 minutes after decreases in segmental wall thickening. Thus, ischemia does not produce ST segment change as promptly or consistently as it does SWMA.

Because two-dimensional echocardiography reliably detects SWMA in animals,[6] numerous studies have been undertaken to define the role of echocardiography in detecting myocardial ischemia in humans. A number of these studies are reviewed to document the superiority of TEE as an intraoperative monitor for myocardial ischemia.

STUDIES IN HUMANS WITH PRECORDIAL ECHOCARDIOGRAPHY

When high-resolution two-dimensional ultrasonographic (echocardiographic) machines became widely available in the late 1970s, echocardiography became a practical tool for the evaluation of patients with ischemic heart disease. For example, Horowitz and colleagues studied 80 consecutive patients within 12 hours of hospital admission for chest pain.[7] Patients with a history of myocardial infarction, valvular heart disease, or cardiomyopathy were excluded. Of the 65 patients with adequate echocardiographic studies, 33 suffered an acute myocardial infarction, and 32 did not. Thirty-one of the 33 patients with acute infarction had SWMA on their initial echocardiogram, but 18 of these

33 had nondiagnostic admission ECGs. Twenty-seven of the 32 patients without acute infarction had normal segmental wall motion. No patient with normal segmental wall motion (0 of 29) suffered a cardiac complication during hospitalization, while 10 of 36 patients with SWMA had complications (severe arrhythmia, recurrent chest pain, heart failure, or death). In this subset of patients, the initial echocardiogram was more sensitive and more specific for the diagnosis of myocardial infarction and prediction of subsequent complications than the initial ECG.

With the advent of percutaneous transluminal coronary angioplasty (PTCA), investigators had an ideal model for evaluation of acute myocardial ischemia in humans. Hauser and colleagues studied the sequence of mechanical, ECG, and clinical effects of PTCA in 18 patients.[8] Interruption of coronary blood flow by inflation of the dilating balloon produced new SWMA in the distribution of the instrumented coronary artery in 86% of the dilations; it did not, however, alter the wall motion when highly collateralized areas of myocardium were involved or when baseline wall motion was absent. The onset of the SWMA began approximately 19 seconds after coronary occlusion and began to normalize 17 seconds after reperfusion. Seven ECG leads were monitored (limb leads, augmented leads, and V_5). ST segment change occurred in 30% of the dilations approximately 30 seconds after coronary artery occlusion. ST changes invariably occurred after the onset of SWMA but usually before the onset of chest pain (39 seconds after occlusion in 41% of dilations). Thus, during PTCA these investigators demonstrated that SWMA invariably precede ECG changes and often occur in their absence.

Most of the customary precordial ECG leads, however, were not used in this study. In contrast, Wohlgelernter and associates used the standard 12-lead ECG in 30 patients who were undergoing PTCA.[9] All patients in this study had a positive exercise treadmill test, an isolated obstructive lesion of the left anterior descending coronary artery without collateral blood supply, normal baseline left ventricular function, and no conduction disturbances or ST segment abnormalities on the ECG that would preclude assessment of ischemia. All patients developed SWMA 10 seconds (on the average) after coronary artery occlusion, and 27 of 30 (90%) developed ST segment change at 22 seconds. Thus, in this carefully selected population who experienced 45 to 90 seconds of complete coronary occlusion, SWMA were an earlier and more sensitive indicator of myocardial ischemia than the 12-lead ECG.

INTRAOPERATIVE STUDIES WITH TRANSESOPHAGEAL ECHOCARDIOGRAPHY

With the introduction in West Germany of a two-dimensional echocardiographic transducer that could be positioned in the esophagus, intraoperative echocardiography became a practical tool for anesthesiologists.[10] Beaupre and associates first reported use of this technique for intraoperative detection of myocardial infarction.[11] After cardiopulmonary bypass, they noted a new anteroseptal SWMA, which persisted until the conclusion of surgery. Within 18 hours after surgery, an anteroseptal myocardial infarction was confirmed by ECG changes.

Subsequently, Smith and associates used TEE in 50 patients who were undergoing coronary artery or major vascular surgery.[12] At predetermined intervals, echocardiograms and multilead ECGs (limb leads, augmented leads, and V_5) were recorded, both of which were evaluated by "blinded" observers. All patients had postoperative ECGs and cardiac isoenzyme studies. Intraoperatively, six patients had ST segment changes diagnostic of myocardial ischemia (greater than or equal to 0.1 mV deviation), while 24 had new SWMA diagnostic of myocardial ischemia (Table 3-1). No patient experienced an ST segment change before or in the absence of a new SWMA. In three of the six patients who experienced ST segment change, the SWMA occurred minutes before the ECG change. Three of the 50 patients suffered intraoperative myocardial infarctions, and all had an SWMA develop and persist until the

TABLE 3-1. Segmental Wall-Motion Scoring System

Wall Motion	Radial Shortening*	Myocardial Thickening†
Normal motion	> 30%	+++
Mild hypokinesia	10%–30%	++
Severe hypokinesia	> 0, < 10%	+
Akinesia	0	0
Dyskinesia	Systolic lengthening	Systolic thinning

*Radial shortening is defined as the decrease in length during systole of an imaginary radius from the endocardium to the center of the left ventricular cavity in the midpapillary muscle short-axis cross section. A floating reference system is used.

†Myocardial thickening is defined as the increase in distance between the endocardial and epicardial borders during systole. Diagnosis of myocardial ischemia requires a worsening of wall motion by at least two classes.

(Adapted from Smith JS, Cahalan MK, Benefiel DJ et al: Intraoperative detection of myocardial ischemia in high risk patients: Electrocardiography versus two dimensional transesophageal echocardiography. Circulation 72:1015, 1985)

end of surgery in the corresponding area of myocardium. Only one of these patients had intraoperative ST segment change diagnostic of ischemia. During the course of surgery, 24 patients had a total of 32 new SWMA. Two patients had baseline hypokinetic segments that subsequently became dyskinetic. The remaining 22 had normal baseline wall motion in a segment that subsequently developed an abnormality. Of these 22, 4 had segmental dyskinesia, 9 segmental akinesia, and 9 severe segmental hypokinesia. Four of the five patients with double-vessel disease had new SWMA, and these changes were in regions of myocardium supplied by the diseased coronary arteries and never in the "risk-free" myocardium. Ten patients without coronary disease were also studied, and none of these patients had ST segment changes or SWMA. In the 50 patients with coronary disease, 97% of the echocardiograms were analyzed, but inadequate resolution or an inappropriate cross section prevented analysis in the other 3%. In contrast, only 86% of the ECGs were analyzed because of the intraoperative onset of bundle-branch block or paced rhythm. Thus, intraoperative SWMA are an earlier and more reliable sign of myocardial ischemia and impending infarction than ST segment change.

In a similar study, in which continuous TEE and 2-lead Holter recordings were used in patients who were undergoing coronary artery surgery, Leung and associates found comparable results.[13] Six of their 50 patients had uninterpretable ST segments, while no patient had an uninterpretable echocardiogram. During simultaneous TEE and ECG monitoring, 56 new SWMA occurred, of which 8 (14%) were accompanied by ST segment change; and 18 ST segment changes occurred, of which 8 (44%) were accompanied by new SWMA, 4 (22%) by equivocal SWMA (decrease of one class in segmental motion, see Table 3-1), and 6 (33%) by no change in segmental wall motion. Hemodynamics were monitored continuously, but rarely did a change of more than 20% in heart rate, systemic blood pressure, or pulmonary artery diastolic pressure accompany the onset of a new SWMA or ST segment change. Six of the 50 patients had major adverse outcomes (two deaths from cardiac causes, three myocardial infarctions, and one ventricular failure). All six of these patients had new SWMA detected after cardiopulmonary bypass that persisted to the conclusion of surgery. Two of the six had new ST segment changes after bypass, and three others had uninterpretable ST segments due to bundle-branch block or ventricular pacing. No patient without a new SWMA that occurred after cardiopulmonary bypass had a major adverse outcome. Thus, myocardial ischemia was detected more frequently with TEE than with ECG, usually in the presence of apparently normal hemodynamics, and new SWMA that persist were important prognostic signs for cardiovascular complications.

These "intraoperative" studies, however, used postoperative interpretations of the echocardiograms. In addition, they did not explore many inherent difficulties in the use of TEE as a monitor for intraoperative myocardial ischemia.

PROBLEMS IN MONITORING MYOCARDIAL ISCHEMIA WITH TRANSESOPHAGEAL ECHOCARDIOGRAPHY

In their patients, Smith and colleagues and Leung and colleagues used TEE to monitor the midpapillary muscle short-axis cross section of the left ventricle (Fig. 3-1). This cross section is readily obtainable with TEE and is the best cross section for intraoperative monitoring for three reasons. First, all three major coronary arteries supply myocardium viewed in this cross section (Fig. 3-2). The right coronary supplies the inferior wall and part of the septum. The left anterior descending supplies part

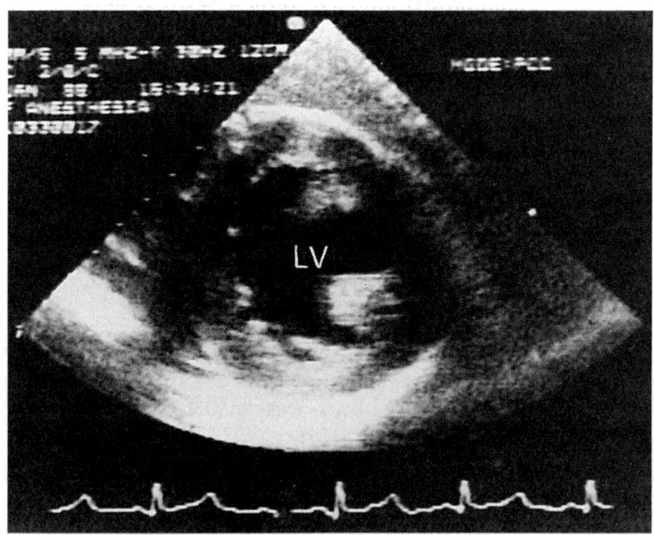

FIGURE 3-1. Short-axis transesophageal echocardiogram at the mid-papillary muscle level. *LV* indicates left ventricular cavity. See *Figure 3-2* for orientation.

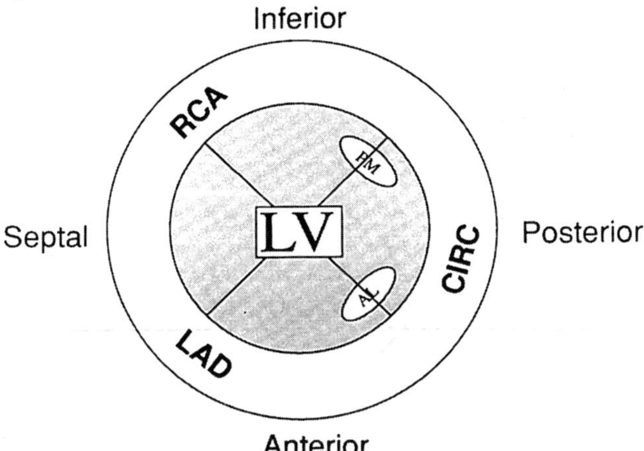

FIGURE 3-2. Diagrammatic short-axis transesophageal echocardiogram at the midpapillary muscle level. *LV* indicates left ventricular cavity; *AL* and *PM*, anterior lateral and posterior medial papillary muscles. The *LV* is divided into 4 segments or walls by two perpendicular lines that bisect the papillary muscles. The walls are by convention named anterior, posterior, septal, and inferior. Coronary blood flow is supplied to these walls as indicated by the left anterior descending coronary artery *(LAD)*, the circumflex coronary artery *(CIRC)*, and the right coronary artery *(RCA)*.

of the septum and anterior wall, while the circumflex artery usually supplies the remainder of the anterior and posterior (free wall) of the left ventricle at this midpapillary muscle level. Second, changes in left ventricular filling cause larger changes in the short-axis dimension than in the long-axis dimension. Thus, changes in filling are more easily appreciated by viewing the short-axis cross section. Third, movement of the probe from its monitoring position at the short-axis, midpapillary muscle level is immediately apparent because the morphology of the papillary muscles changes as they extend from their origins in the wall of the ventricle to their insertions into the chordae. Changes in filling and contraction are assessed during surgery relative to the initial echocardiogram obtained after induction of anesthesia, and, to make such evaluations valid, the same cross section must be viewed.

However, ischemia confined to the right ventricle, base, or apex of the left ventricle will be missed if only the midpapillary muscle cross section is monitored. This fact may explain in part why Leung and associates found six episodes of significant ST segment change unaccompanied by new SWMA. One solution is to frequently reposition the probe to view other cross sections; however, this practice is impractical when one anesthesiologist is responsible for both patient care and TEE monitoring. Another potential solution is provided by a new biplane transesophageal probe, which has two transducers with their ultrasound beams oriented at right angles to each other. With this probe ideally positioned, the anesthesiologist can immediately switch from the midpapillary muscle short-axis cross section to a long-axis cross section and view portions of the left ventricular base and apex (Fig. 3-3). However, both cross sections cannot be viewed simultaneously in real time, and no studies yet available document an improved rate of ischemia detection with this new probe.

Even when an area of myocardium is clearly in view, its segmental contraction can be difficult to evaluate if the entire heart rotates or translates markedly during systole or if discoordinated contraction occurs due to bundle-branch block or ventricular pacing. Consequently, a valid system for assessing SWMA must first compensate for global motion of the heart (usually done by a "floating" frame of reference) and then evaluate both regional endocardial motion and myocardial thickening. Unfortunately, no automated wall motion analysis system available has proven adequate for TEE images. Interpretation of septal motion is most often confounded by discoordinated contraction. When the septum is viable and nonischemic, it appreciably thickens during systole, although its inward motion may begin slightly before or after inward motion of the other walls of the ventricle. Thus, new SWMA can be detected during bundle-branch block, ventricular pacing, and marked global movements of the heart, but not by assessment of endocardial motion alone.

However, are all SWMA indicative of myocardial ischemia or infarction? Clearly, they are not. Because of biologic differences in normal patients, not all hearts contract normally, and not all parts of the same heart contract to the same degree.[14] However, an acute decrease or cessation of segmental contraction, for example a new SWMA during surgery (Figs. 3-4 and 3-5), is almost certainly due to myocardial ischemia. One exception to this rule is myocardial stunning, or prolonged, postischemic ventricular dysfunction.[15] When ischemia has been prolonged, full restoration of blood flow may occur minutes to hours before return of normal segmental contraction. Does a new SWMA detected immediately after bypass represent inadequate revascularization and ongoing ischemia or stunned myocardium from inadequate

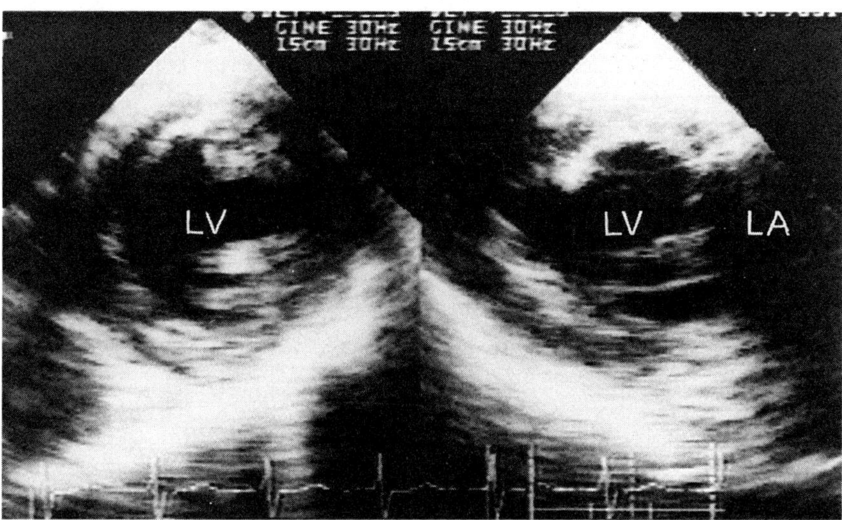

FIGURE 3-3. Short-axis *(left)* and long-axis *(right)* transesophageal echocardiograms. These images were produced without repositioning the biplane probe, but by switching electronically from one of its transducers to another. The structures between left atrial cavity *(LA)* and left ventricular cavity *(LV)* are mitral valve and chordae tendineae.

cooling during bypass? Inadequate revascularization may require placement of additional grafts, while stunned myocardium requires only supportive measures until its function returns. Unfortunately, echocardiographic contrast agents capable of readily delineating myocardial blood flow are not yet clinically available. Therefore, when this clinical dilemma is encountered, graft status is reevaluated and the new SWMA watched for signs of improvement. If worsening occurs, if graft status is questionable, or if hemodynamics are tenuous, then additional revascularization is provided if possible.

Another conceivable cause of acute SWMA is unmasking areas of scarring by changes in afterload. For instance, a marked increase in blood pressure might retard contraction in an already damaged segment of myocardium more than in a normal segment. Three observations make this explanation unlikely for the acute SWMA reported in the studies above. First, only marked changes in segmental contraction were taken as indicative of ischemia (see Table 3-1). It is hard to imagine that a sudden increase in afterload would cause one segment to cease or nearly cease contracting in the absence of changes in the other

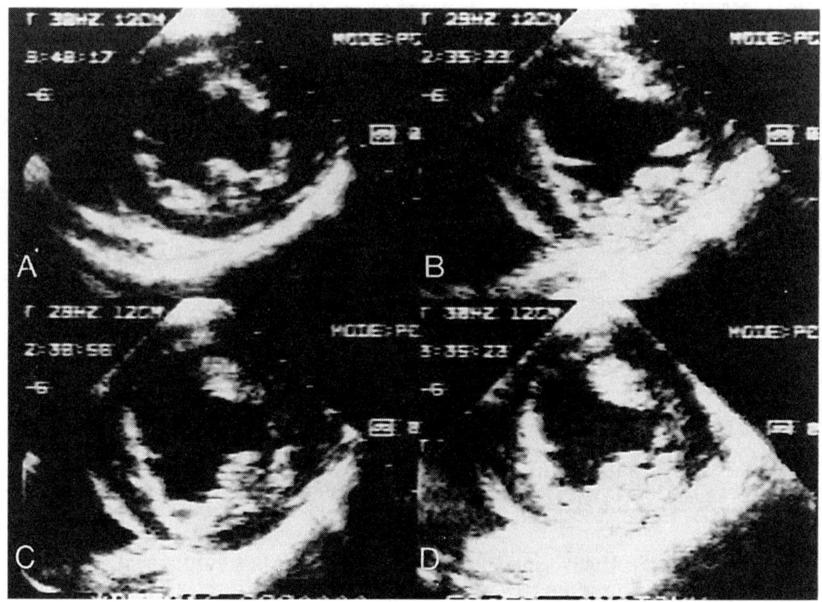

FIGURE 3-4. Four short-axis, end-diastolic transesophageal echocardiograms recorded at: *A,* after induction of anesthesia; *B,* immediately after cardiopulmonary bypass; *C,* approximately 10 minutes after cardiopulmonary bypass; and *D,* after placement of an additional coronary bypass graft. See *Figure 3-5* for additional details. Orientation of images is the same as in *Figure 3-2.*

segments. Second, neither group of investigators found any consistent correlation between hemodynamic aberrations and new SWMA. In general, anesthesiologists prevent marked changes in loading conditions. Third, the vast majority of new SWMA occurred in segments of myocardium with normal contraction at baseline (after induction of anesthesia). Thus, acute changes in left ventricular loading probably require an intervention by the anesthesiologist and can cause myocardial ischemia but alone are not an explanation for new SWMA.

Tethering, or systolic dysfunction of nonischemic myocardium adjacent to ischemic or infarcted myocardium, is also commonly mentioned as another cause of "artifactual" SWMA. Tethering probably accounts for the consistent overestimation of infarct size by echocardiography when compared to post mortem studies. However, Force and colleagues used an improved analysis system and found that segmental contraction is normal to within 1 cm of the ischemic area.[16] Thus, tethering may actually help the intraoperative detection of myocardial isch-

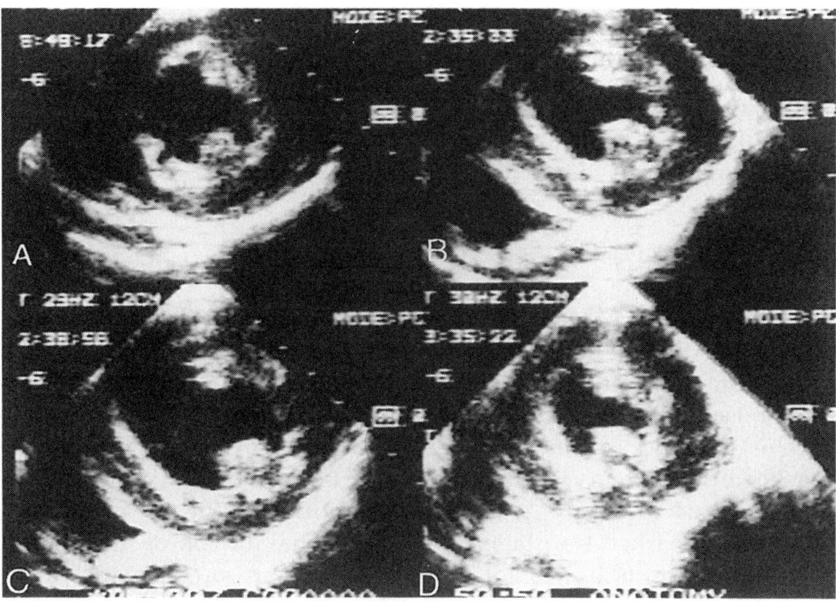

FIGURE 3-5. The corresponding four short-axis, end-systolic transesophageal echocardiograms recorded at the same intervals as shown in *Figure 3-4.* Notice that septal motion and thickening are normal in *A* and *D,* but akinetic in *B,* and dyskinetic in *C.*

emia by making a new SWMA involve an area of myocardium slightly larger than the true area of ischemia. Tethering does not create new SWMA in the absence of acute myocardial ischemia.

Even if TEE can be refined to image all new SWMA, anesthesiologists must recognize them in real time to institute appropriate, timely therapy. Clements and de Bruijn found that after 20 minutes of instruction, 53 clinicians correctly identified 95% of SWMA replayed for them from videotape.[17] However, Saada and colleagues reported a much lower recognition rate when anesthesiologists were asked to evaluate segmental wall motion in real time while they were administering anesthesia.[18] In this latter study of 29 patients, six new SWMA (worsening of segmental function by at least two classes) occurred, and neither group of anesthesiologists (resident or faculty) recognized three of them. In the three other ischemic episodes, the quad-screen system used allowed the juxtapositioning of the baseline echocardiogram (the images from one cardiac cycle played continuously) and subsequent echocardiograms on the same video screen. With this technique, both group of anesthesiologists (resident and faculty) recognized two of the ischemic episodes, and one group recognized the third. Clearly, new SWMA can be missed by the anesthesiologist if recall of baseline wall motion is inadequate. Quad-screen systems are commercially available and definitely help to recognize SWMA as well as changes in global ejection and filling.

CONCLUSION

In animal models and in human studies in the catheterization laboratory and in the operating room, echocardiographically detected SWMA have been proven to be earlier and more sensitive indicators of myocardial ischemia than ECG-detected ST segment changes or acute changes in hemodynamics. In addition, when new SWMA persist to the conclusion of surgery, myocardial infarction or other cardiovascular complications are likely to occur. Detection of SWMA can be confounded by marked translational and rotational motion of the heart or by incoordinate contraction of the ventricle during bundle-branch block or ventricular pacing. However, myocardial thickening during systole is a hallmark of nonischemic, viable myocardium and can be assessed even in the presence of these confounding effects. Clearly, TEE has already become a powerful research tool for anesthesiologists and is likely to become a clinical tool in many other centers in part because of its superior ability to detect myocardial ischemia.

References

1. Tennant R, Wiggers CJ: The effect of coronary occlusion on myocardial infarction. Am J Physiol 112:351, 1935
2. Forrester JS, Wyatt HL, da Luz PL, Tyberg JV, Diamond GA, Swan HJC: Functional significance of regional ischemic contraction abnormalities. Circulation 54:64, 1976
3. Vatner SF: Correlation between acute reductions in myocardial blood flow and function in conscious dogs. Circ Res 47:201, 1980
4. Waters DD, da Luz P, Wyatt HL, Swan HJ, Forrester JS: Early changes in regional and global left ventricular function induced by graded reductions in regional coronary perfusion. Am J Cardiol 39:537, 1977
5. Battler A, Froelicher VF, Gallagher KP, Kemper WS, Ross J Jr: Dissociation between regional myocardial dysfunction and ECG changes during ischemia in the conscious dog. Circulation 62:735, 1980
6. Pandian NG, Kerber RE: Two dimensional echocardiography in experimental coronary stenosis. I. Sensitivity and specificity in detecting transient myocardial dyskinesis: Comparison with sonomicrometers. Circulation 66:597, 1982

7. Horowitz RS, Morganroth J, Parrotto C, Chen CC, Soffer J, Pauletto FJ: Immediate diagnosis of acute myocardial infarction by two-dimensional echocardiography. Circulation 65:323, 1982
8. Hauser AM, Gangadharan V, Ramos RG, Gordon S, Timmis GC: Sequence of mechanical, electrocardiographic and clinical effects of repeated coronary artery occlusion in human beings: Echocardiographic observations during coronary angioplasty. J Am Coll Cardiol 5:193, 1985
9. Wohlgelernter D, Jaffe CC, Cabin HS, Yeatman LA, Cleman M: Silent ischemia during coronary occlusion produced by balloon inflation: Relation to regional myocardial dysfunction. J Am Coll Cardiol 10:491, 1987
10. Schluter M, Langenstein BA, Polster J et al: Transesophageal cross sectional echocardiography with a phased array transducer system: Technique and initial clinical results. Br Heart J 48:67, 1982
11. Beaupre PN, Kremer PF, Cahalan MK, Lurz FW, Schiller NB: Intraoperative detection of changes in left ventricular segmental wall motion by transesophageal two-dimensional echocardiography. Am Heart J 107: 1021, 1984
12. Smith JS, Cahalan MK, Benefiel DJ et al: Intraoperative detection of myocardial ischemia in high risk patients: Electrocardiography versus two dimensional transesophageal echocardiography. Circulation 72:1015, 1985
13. Leung JM, O'Kelley B, Browner WS, Tubau J, Hollenberg M, Mangano DT: Prognostic importance of postbypass regional wall-motion abnormalities in patients undergoing coronary artery bypass graft surgery. Anesthesiology 71:16, 1989
14. Pandian NG, Skorton DJ, Collins SM, Falsetti HL, Burke ER, Kerber RE: Heterogeneity of left ventricular segmental wall motion thickening and excursion in 2-dimensional echocardiograms of normal human subjects. Am J Cardiol 51:1677, 1983
15. Braunwald E, Kloner RA: The stunned myocardium: Prolonged, postischemic ventricular dysfunction. Circulation 66:1146, 1982
16. Force T, Kemper A, Perkins L, Gilfoil M, Cohen C, Parisi AF: Overestimation of infarct size by quantitative two-dimensional echocardiography: The role of tethering and of analytic procedures. Circulation 73:1360, 1986
17. Clements FM, de Bruijn NP: Perioperative evaluation of regional wall motion by transesophageal two-dimensional echocardiography. Anesth Analg 66:249, 1987
18. Saada M, Cahalan MK, Lee E, Ionescu P, Schiller NB: Real-time evaluation of echocardiograms. Anesthesiology 71:A344, 1989

Jacqueline M. Leung
Nelson B. Schiller
Dennis T. Mangano

4 Assessment of Left Ventricular Function Using Two-Dimensional Transesophageal Echocardiography

Two-dimensional transesophageal echocardiography (TEE) is a new imaging technique that is gaining increasing popularity as an intraoperative monitor of left ventricular (LV) function. Because of the possibility of assessing LV function serially and even continuously with little risk to the patient, intraoperative TEE monitoring is particularly useful in monitoring patients with coronary artery disease, who are at risk for developing intraoperative ventricular dysfunction. Previous reports have used this technique to examine a number of indices of LV function, including regional wall motion and myocardial thickening, preload, afterload, and wall stress. This review discusses the results of these studies, as well as the implications and limitations of their findings.

IMAGING CARDIAC CHAMBERS FROM THE ESOPHAGUS

With the development of a phased-array transducer adapted for transesophageal use, imaging of the heart posteriorly from the esophagus

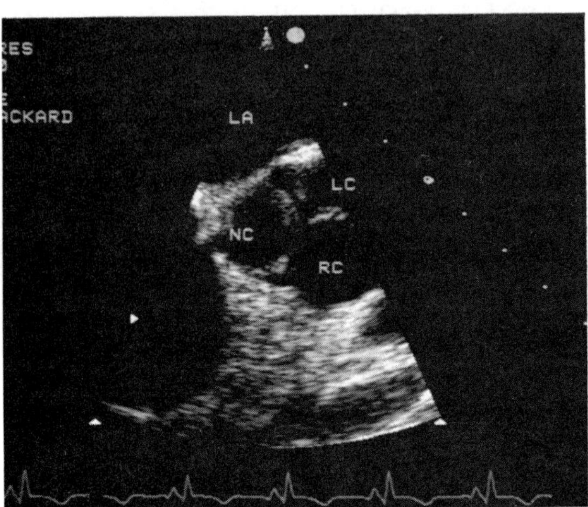

FIGURE 4-1. The aortic valve view showing an image at the level of the aortic root. The three aortic cusps are outlined. The right ventricular outflow tract is imaged anteriorly, and part of the left atrium *(LA)* is imaged immediately posterior to the aortic root. *LC,* left coronary cusp; *NC,* noncoronary cusp; *RC,* right coronary cusp.

became possible.[1] Because of its proximity to the heart, sound waves emitted from the esophageal transducer only have to pass through the esophageal wall and the pericardium before reaching the heart. Thus, less image distortion is found from the ribs and the lungs. Imaging from the esophagus provides better images than those from precordial imaging.[1] Furthermore, because of the stability of the transducer and its unobtrusive location, TEE is most suited for continuous monitoring for extended periods of time without interference with the surgical field.

The usual method for intraoperative TEE monitoring is as follows: after anesthetic induction and intubation of the patient's trachea, the transducer is inserted orally and advanced into the esophagus 30 to 40 cm from the incisors to obtain the *aortic root view* (Fig. 4-1). If resistance is met during the initial insertion, chin lift or direct laryngoscopy is used to facilitate insertion. At times, deflation of the cuff of the endotracheal tube is necessary. Morphologic aspects of the aortic valve can be evaluated using this view. With further advancement and clockwise rotation of the gastroscope, the left side of the heart is transected in a plane oblique to the LV long axis (Fig. 4-2). The left atrium (LA), the mitral valve, the ventricular septum, the LV outflow tract, the lateral LV wall,

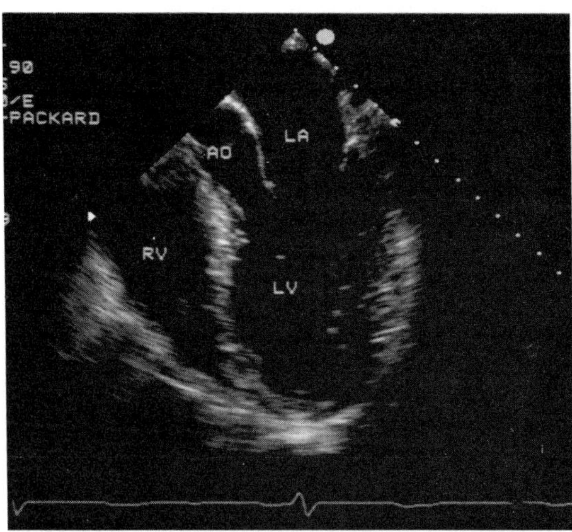

FIGURE 4-2. The long-axis view showing the left side of the heart with part of the right ventricle. Both mitral leaflets are outlined. *LV,* left ventricle; *AO,* aorta; *RV,* right ventricle; *LA,* left atrium.

as well as a portion of the right ventricle are imaged. The transducer is then advanced beyond the gastroesophageal junction, and, using the controls on the gastroscope, the transducer can be flexed behind the inferior wall of the LV to obtain a *short-axis view* at the midpapillary level (Fig. 4-3). This view is characterized by a circular shape of the LV cavity, with the posteromedial papillary muscle imaged at the 11-o'clock position, and the anterolateral papillary muscle at the 7-o'clock position.

At the San Francisco Veterans Administration Medical Center, more than 700 patients who were undergoing cardiac and noncardiac surgery have been studied using continuous TEE as a monitor of myocardial ischemia. More than 3000 hours of continuous TEE data have been collected and analyzed. Typically, the short-axis view is monitored continuously throughout the operation and for as long as 12 to 16 hours, extending into the intensive care unit. When combined with the experience from the Moffitt-Long Hospital at the University of California, San Francisco, more than 3000 patients have been clinically monitored with TEE. No major complication has occurred. Generally, complications from intraoperative TEE monitoring are rare if precautions are taken to exclude patients with a history of dysphagia, esophageal disease, or prior esophageal surgery.

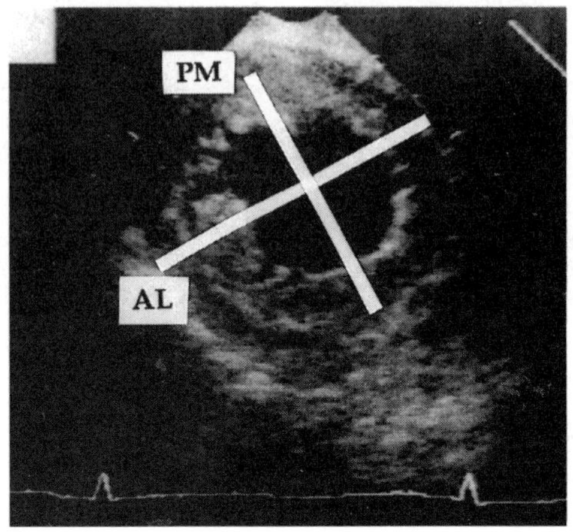

Grade
0 Normal
1 Mild hypokinesis
2 Severe hypokinesis
3 Akinesis
4 Dyskinesis

Criteria:
i) change of grade ≥ 2
ii) wall motion score

FIGURE 4-3. The short-axis view showing a cross-section of the left ventricle at the level of the papillary muscles. The left ventricle appears circular in shape. *PM,* postero-medial papillary muscles; *AL,* antero-lateral papillary muscles.

ASSESSMENT OF REGIONAL LEFT VENTRICULAR FUNCTION

Tennant and Wiggers were the first to describe how coronary artery ligation resulted in an immediate cessation of contraction of cardiac muscle supplied by this vessel.[2] The affected area appears cyanotic, dilated, and bulging. These immediate effects occur and develop simultaneously with the rise in myocardial lactate that is detected in the venous drainage of an ischemic region.[3] Without oxygen, the production of high-energy phosphates fails, leading to anaerobic metabolism and regional lactic acidosis. Ischemia further reduces the release of calcium from the sarcolemma, the sarcoplasmic reticulum, or both, making less calcium available to the contractile sites.[4] The earliest physiologic changes following experimental coronary artery ligation are changes in myocardial wall thickening, followed by changes in the endocardial electrocardiography (ECG) and then the surface ECG.[5]

Previous reports have used both semiquantitative and quantitative two-dimensional TEE to assess regional LV function. A summary of the most relevant previous intraoperative studies that used TEE to assess LV function is provided in Table 4-1.[6–22] In an early study of 24 patients who were undergoing aortic reconstruction, Roizen and colleagues reported frequent regional wall motion abnormalities (RWMA) in patients with aortic occlusion at the supraceliac level.[8] These changes were not always detected by traditional monitoring devices, such as pulmonary artery pressure monitoring. In fact, the pulmonary artery wedge pressure was always within the normal range, except for transient increase in two of twelve patients who were undergoing aortic occlusion at the supraceliac level. Subsequent studies by Topol and associates[9] and Koolen and associates[14] used intermittent TEE to study patients who were undergoing coronary artery bypass graft (CABG) surgery and found that regional ventricular function frequently improved immediately after myocardial revascularization. These findings, however, should be interpreted with caution. Both studies used an off-line computer-assisted method to quantitate regional thickening[9] and regional fractional area change.[14] The end-diastolic and end-systolic endocardial borders were outlined using a computer-assisted contouring system. As previously observed, peak systolic shortening occurs variably, depending on the ventricular segment under consideration.[23] Since asynchrony is not infrequent following cardiopulmonary bypass, assessment by quantitative wall thickening alone can overestimate or underestimate regional function if only end-diastolic and end-systolic images are analyzed.[24–26] Furthermore, in the study by Topol and associates, epicardial borders were also traced and observer bias can be

TABLE 4-1. Previous Studies That Used TEE to Assess LV Function

Author	Year	No. of Patients	Type of Operations	Parameters Measured
Beaupre et al[6]	1983	32	Renal, aortic, CABG	EDA, ESA
Roizen et al[7]	1983	3	Pheochromocytoma	EDA, ESA, FAC
Roizen et al[8]	1984	24	Aortic reconstruction	EDA, ESA, RWMA
Topol et al[9]	1984	20	CABG	Regional thickening
Smith et al[10]	1985	50	CABG/vascular	RWMA
Konstadt et al[11]	1986	10	CABG	EDA, ESA, FAC
Shively et al[12]	1986	57	CABG	RWMA/prediction of MI
Gewertz et al[13]	1987	49	Vascular	RWMA
Koolen et al[14]	1987	30	CABG	Regional area EF
Abel et al[15]	1987	11	CABG	EDA, ESA, FAC, RWMA, systolic wall thickening
Slavik et al[16]	1988	7	CABG	EDA, ESA, FAC, RWMA
London et al[17]	1988	95	Vascular/major vasc	RWMA
O'Kelly et al[18]	1988	6	CABG	LV contractility
Smith et al[19]	1988	60	Carotid	LV end-systolic wall stress, fiber shortening, RWMA
Leung et al[20]	1989	50	CABG	RWMA/prediction of adverse outcomes
Saada et al[21]	1989	13	Cardiac/vascular	RWMA
Leung et al[22]	1989	84	CABG	RWMA/anesthetic effects

CABG, coronary artery bypass grafting; EDA, end-diastolic area; ESA, end-systolic area; FAC, fractional area change; RWMA, regional wall motion abnormalities; MI, myocardial infection; EF, ejection fraction; LV left ventricular.

introduced since resolution of epicardial borders is frequently poor.[9] Abel and colleagues studied 11 patients who were undergoing CABG surgery and found that measurements of systolic wall thickening correlated poorly with visual regional wall motion analysis.[15] In addition, intraobserver variability demonstrated a marked degree of random error.

Another controversy in quantitative TEE is the selection of a frame of reference for the computerized comparison between the end-diastolic and end-systolic contours. The heart rotates and translates in the thoracic cavity during the cardiac cycle. These cardiac movements can either be ignored or corrected, depending on whether an external (fixed) reference or an internal (floating axis) reference system is used. Previous studies have supported both the fixed reference[27,28] and the floating axis reference system.[29,30] Two recent quantitative intraoperative TEE studies have used the floating axis reference, center of mass system.[14,16] If a dyskinetic wall segment bulges outward during systole, the center of mass moves toward the abnormally contracting segment. Realignment of this center with the end-diastolic center makes the dyskinetic segment appear to be moving normally while the normal segment appears hypokinetic or akinetic. The controversy over reference system, therefore, remains unresolved and awaits further investigation.

In contrast, a semiquantitative way of analyzing RWMA has been used at the University of California, San Francisco. The short-axis, cross-sectional image is divided into four segments, using the papillary muscles as guides (Fig. 4-4). The wall motion of each of the four segments are graded to be normal or to have mild hypokinesia, severe hypokinesia, akinesia, or dyskinesia. A segment is judged to be isch-

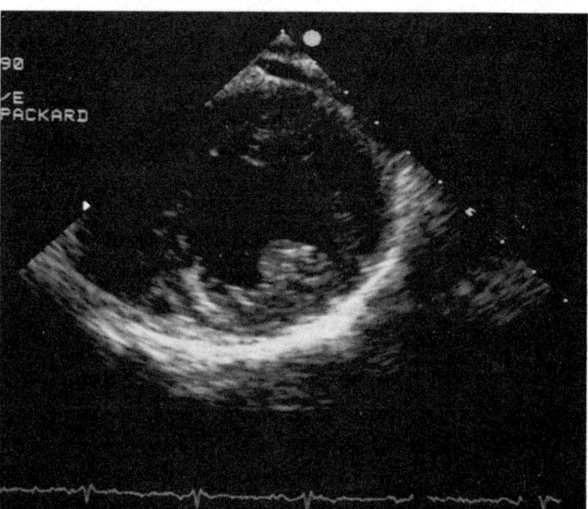

FIGURE 4-4. Semiquantitative analysis of regional wall motion abnormalities at the level of the short-axis view. The left ventricular short-axis view is left-right inverted in this figure as compared to figure 4-3.

emic when wall motion of any segment worsens by two or more grades. Using such a grading system, Smith and colleagues studied 50 patients who were undergoing either vascular or CABG surgery.[10] At predetermined intervals, echocardiograms and multiple-lead ECGs were recorded and evaluated by "blinded" investigators. Intraoperatively, 24 of the 50 patients had new RWMA, whereas only six had ST segment changes. All patients with ST segment changes also had new RWMA. Of the four patients who had perioperative myocardial infarctions, three had persistent intraoperative RWMA and one had a transient intraoperative RWMA, whereas, only one patient had ST segment changes. This study is the first to demonstrate the greater sensitivity of TEE vs. ECG for the intraoperative detection of myocardial ischemia.

Since RWMA are sensitive indicators of myocardial ischemia, the use of TEE may have substantial impact on the early detection and characterization of perioperative myocardial ischemia in patients who are undergoing CABG surgery. To evaluate the prognostic importance of RWMA, Leung and associates prospectively studied 50 patients who were undergoing elective CABG surgery, using continuous TEE, ECG (2-lead Holter), and hemodynamic measurements during the prebypass, postbypass, and early postoperative intensive care unit (ICU) periods.[20] Echocardiographic and ECG evidence of ischemia during each of the three periods was characterized and related to adverse clinical outcomes (postoperative myocardial infarction, ventricular failure, and cardiac death). A unique feature of this study is that clinicians were "blinded" to both the TEE and ECG information. To "blind" the echocardiographic readers, the temporal sequence of the echocardiographic samples were scrambled before analysis. The prevalence of myocardial ischemia during the perioperative periods was prebypass, 20% (TEE) vs. 7% (ECG); postbypass, 36% (TEE) vs. 25% (ECG); and ICU, 25% (TEE) vs. 16% (ECG). Neither prebypass TEE ischemia nor ECG ischemia that occurred in any of the three periods predicted adverse outcome. In contrast, postbypass TEE ischemia was predictive of outcome: 6 out of 18 patients with postbypass TEE ischemia had adverse outcomes vs. 0 out of 32 without TEE ischemia. Seventy-three percent of the echocardiographic ischemic episodes occurred without acute change (plus or minus 20% of control) in heart rate, systemic arterial pressure, or pulmonary arterial pressure. Intraoperative TEE, therefore, appears unique in its ability to identify both patients that are at high risk and the highest risk periods for myocardial ischemia.

In a study of 95 high-risk patients (those with coronary artery disease or two or more risk factors) who were undergoing noncardiac surgery, London and associates used continuous TEE and continuous 12-

lead ECG to characterize the incidence of intraoperative myocardial ischemia.[17] They found a relatively high incidence (33%) with TEE of new intraoperative RWMA in these patients. Furthermore, these changes occurred more frequently than ECG ischemia. This study is still under way, and its results will elucidate the role of TEE as a clinical monitoring tool in noncardiac surgery.

The ability of TEE to detect early changes in myocardial ischemia provides a unique opportunity for anesthesiologists to determine the effects of anesthetics on the myocardium. In a preliminary report on 84 patients, the effects of isoflurane, a potent inhalational agent that has been shown to cause coronary-artery steal in an animal model, were compared to sufentanil, a highly lipid soluble, potent narcotic, in patients who were undergoing elective CABG surgery.[22] Patients were monitored continuously at the midpapillary level with TEE after being randomized to receive either sufentanil or isoflurane. Heart rate and systolic blood pressure were rigorously controlled within plus or minus 20% of preoperative baseline. Using strict hemodynamic control and a sensitive measure of myocardial ischemia, TEE, the overall incidence of prebypass ischemia was 21%. Isoflurane was associated with a similar incidence of moderate to severe TEE ischemic episodes as sufentanil. In this setting, intraoperative TEE offers new information that is essential to our understanding of anesthetic effects on the heart.

Both quantitative and semiquantitative TEE analyses, however, are tedious. These methods require knowledge and expertise in echocardiographic interpretation. The observer has to examine each segment in turn for wall thickening and inward motion during systole. In addition, semiquantitative assessment can be subjective if the observers do not adhere to strict guidelines established for regional wall motion analysis. Accuracy and consistency of echocardiographic interpretation require frequent determination of both intraobserver and interobserver variabilities. A recent study by Saada and colleagues examines the validity of real-time intraoperative evaluation of TEE. Anesthesia residents (with minimal TEE experience) and faculty anesthesiologists (with more than 50 cases) were asked to evaluate intraoperatively regional wall motion in real time.[21] The TEE short-axis views were simultaneously recorded on videotapes for subsequent evaluation by two independent, experienced observers. Residents correctly identified 97.2% of normal wall motion, and faculty members, 98.6%. Of the segments with abnormal wall motion detected by the expert readers, residents were able to detect 61.5% and faculty members, 77%. The experienced readers disagreed on 5% of the segments (normal vs. mild hypokinesia). Three episodes of ischemia (change of grade greater than or equal to 2) were detected by the expert readers; one was detected by the faculty members and none by the residents. Thus, even trained observers can miss intraoperative ischemic events. Real-time intraoperative use of TEE for accurately detecting ischemia, therefore, is complex and requires a significant amount of echocardiographic training. Devices that allow the display of two simultaneous images (control and real-time) in cine-loop should help increase the sensitivity of ischemia detection in the intraoperative setting.

ASSESSMENT OF GLOBAL LEFT VENTRICULAR FUNCTION

Preload

Left ventricular preload or the volume of blood at end-diastole is determined by the intraventricular volume. In the intact heart, the preload of the LV can be measured as the LV end-diastolic volume (LVEDV). The LVEDV is difficult to measure clinically and is usually estimated by measurement of the mean left atrial pressure or pulmonary capillary wedge pressure. Conditions that decrease ventricular compliance and mitral valve dysfunction alter the pressure-volume relationship, making assessment of preload difficult. Transesophageal echocardiography has been used extensively to measure the LV end-diastolic area as an approximation of LV volume. Typically, endocardial and epicardial borders at end-diastole and end-systole are traced. End-diastole is indicated by the peak of the R wave, and end-systole is defined as the smallest systolic endocardial area. The fractional area change (FAC), which provides an estimate of ejection fraction, is defined using the calculation in Equation 4-1.

$$\text{FAC (\%)} = \frac{\text{End-Diastolic Area} - \text{End-Systolic Area}}{\text{End-Diastolic Area}} \times 100 \qquad (4\text{-}1)$$

Konstadt and associates studied 10 patients who were undergoing CABG surgery with TEE. He monitored the short-axis LV areas at the level of the papillary muscles and demonstrated a close correlation between TEE and on-heart echocardiographic measurements of end-diastolic area, end-systolic area, and ejection fraction area.[11] Abel and colleagues confirmed these findings in 11 patients scheduled for CABG surgery and concluded that measurements of LV area and FAC obtained intraoperatively with TEE were highly reproducible.[15] However, volume estimation that uses the single short-axis area is potentially inaccurate because TEE monitoring is only two-dimensional: the TEE transducer cannot always be angled to produce a true long-axis view to allow direct measurement of LV length. The clinical and research application of biplane transducers in assessing volume is being investigated.

Despite these limitations, TEE has been shown to provide consistent estimates of changes in LV volume. Beaupre and colleagues studied 32 patients who were undergoing renal transplantation, aortic reconstruction, or CABG surgery and found a high correlation (91%) between echocardiographic estimate of cardiac output ([LVESA − LVEDA] times heart rate) and cardiac output by thermodilution.[6] In contrast, a change in pulmonary artery occlusion pressure predicted a similar change in LVEDA in only 23% of the patients. Hence, in situations where LV compliance is altered, TEE may provide a better estimate of LV volume than routine hemodynamic monitoring. The usefulness of preload estimation from TEE recently was compared to other routinely obtainable hemodynamic parameters in predicting hypovolemia in 139 patients who were undergoing elective CABG surgery.[31] It was found that the appearance of low cardiac volume on TEE was infrequently preceded by any acute alteration in hemodynamic parameters. Overall, only 20% of the low LV volume episodes were associated with increased (greater than 10%) heart rate; with decreased systolic blood pressure, 21%; diastolic blood pressure, 25%; pulmonary artery diastolic pressure, 16%; and central venous pressure, 12%. Therefore, routine hemodynamic measurements appear to be insensitive measures of low LV volume compared to TEE.

Afterload, Wall Stress, Contractility

One of the major determinants of myocardial oxygen demand is wall stress, which is directly related to afterload (a function of LV size and arterial blood pressure). Clinically, afterload is estimated from the systolic blood pressure and systemic vascular resistance. Two-dimensional TEE in combination with ventricular pressure measurements can provide a more accurate measure of wall stress since LV diameter and thickness can be estimated. Reichek and associates found that systolic wall stress estimates calculated using cuff systolic blood pressure correlated closely with estimates made from angiographic parameters and

LV pressures.[32] End-systolic wall stress (ESWS) can be calculated as shown in Equation 4-2,

$$\text{ESWS} = 1.332 \times \frac{Pd}{4h(1 + h/d)} \times 10^3 \text{ dyne/cm}^2 \qquad (4\text{-}2)$$

where P indicates peak intra-arterial pressure or LV end-systolic pressure; d, internal diameter of the ventricle; and h, average wall thickness of the myocardial shell.[33]

Patients with severe coronary artery disease often have compromised ventricular function, which makes them more vulnerable to the acute changes in afterload. Roizen and associates found that with supraceliac occlusion of the aorta, mean systemic arterial pressure increased 54% and was accompanied by an increase in end-systolic area of 69%.[8] Occlusion of the aorta more distally was accompanied by only a minor increase in mean arterial pressure and end-systolic area. Although wall stress was not calculated, it is likely that a marked increase occurred during supraceliac aortic occlusion. A recent report by Smith and associates examined the effects of anesthetic technique on the incidence of TEE ischemia in 60 patients who were undergoing carotid endarterectomy.[19] The patients were randomly assigned to receive halothane or isoflurane (with nitrous oxide) at low concentrations or at higher concentrations (with phenylephrine to support blood pressure). The patients who received high anesthetic concentrations with phenylephrine had a threefold greater incidence of myocardial ischemia than did the patients who received light anesthesia given to maintain similar systolic blood pressures and stump pressures. In addition, although blood pressures were similar, the patients who received a higher concentration of anesthetic plus phenylephrine had a higher wall stress, regardless of the choice of anesthetic agent. Thus, afterload estimation (wall stress) using TEE measurements provides information not routinely obtainable from systolic blood pressure measurements.

Another use of TEE has been the intraoperative estimation of LV contractility. The relationship between meridional stress and LV diameter may be an important load-independent index of myocardial contractile state.[32,34,35] In a group of six patients who were undergoing CABG surgery, O'Kelly and associates measured LV contractility by manipulation of afterload using phenylephrine and nitroprusside infusions.[18] Under general anesthesia, before CABG surgery, measurements were made at baseline and at postventricular ectopic beats with afterload manipulation. The end-systolic area and end-systolic meridional stress correlations were found to be linear. Furthermore, the slope of the relationship was sensitive to changes in LV contractility. Thus, intraoperative measurement of LV contractility is feasible using echocardiographically derived parameters.

LIMITATIONS AND FUTURE APPLICATION

Regional Wall Motion Assessment Using Only Single Plane Transesophageal Echocardiography

A significant percentage of wall motion abnormalities can be detected using the single-plane, short-axis view, but abnormalities that occur in other localized regions, such as the cardiac apex, are not in view.[36–38] Manipulation of the transducer to record multiple views is impractical and introduces errors. Systolic thinning would be a more sensitive indicator,[38] but precise quantitation of the degree of thinning is a limitation (epicardial dropout). Multiple-view transducers are not commercially available, but the research and development of such devices are under way.

Changes in Loading Conditions and Contractility

Regional wall motion abnormalities detected by TEE may have ischemic or nonischemic etiologies. While many factors, such as changes in contractility, preload, afterload, or mechanical tethering of nonischemic myocardium adjacent to ischemic regions,[39] can induce RWMA, evidence suggests only major conduction abnormalities, such as left bundle-branch block, are of major concern. Previous work using intraoperative TEE demonstrated: 1) a strong correlation between intraoperative RWMA and anatomic and physiologic measures of ischemia and areas at risk;[20,40,41] 2) a relationship between RWMA and adverse outcomes;[20] and 3) a relationship between the location of RWMA and the location of myocardial infarction.[20]

Quantitative, Semiquantitative, and Real-Time Assessment of Left Ventricular Function

The limitations of each of these techniques have been outlined previously. The future of intraoperative TEE may lie in the development of on-line quantitative information. Before that is available, extensive training in echocardiographic interpretation is essential for accurate use of this technology.

CONCLUSION

The introduction of intraoperative two-dimensional TEE has provided valuable information for the clinical assessment of LV function. The clinical and research applications of intraoperative TEE, although still at an early stage, have shown promise. The detection of RWMA, which are sensitive indicators of myocardial ischemia, identifies patients who may be at risk for adverse clinical outcome. Early detection of intraoperative myocardial ischemia may aid in the initiation of an aggressive therapy and reversal of such changes before permanent damage to the myocardium occurs. Echocardiographically derived parameters provide accurate estimates of preload, afterload, and LV contractility. The detection of RWMA and the estimation of preload, afterload, and contractility no doubt enhance our ability to assess the effects of surgery and anesthesia on ventricular function. Further advances in technology combined with continuing training and dialogue among its users—anesthesiologists, cardiologists, and surgeons alike—will result no doubt in a more widespread intraoperative use, hopefully leading to significant improvement in patient care.

References

1. Schluter M, Langenstein BA, Polster J et al: Transesophageal cross-sectional echocardiography with a phased array transducer system: Technique and initial clinical results. Br Heart J 48:67, 1982
2. Tennant R, Wiggers CJ: The effect of coronary occlusion on myocardial contraction. Am J Physiol 112:351, 1935
3. Massie BM, Botvinick EH, Brundage BH, Greenberg B, Shames D, Gelberg H: Relationship of regional myocardial perfusion to segmental wall motion: A physiologic basis for understanding the presence and reversibility of asynergy. Circulation 58:1154, 1978
4. Katz AM: Effects of ischemia on the contractile processes of heart muscle. Am J Cardiol 32:456, 1973
5. Battler A, Froelicher VF, Gallagher KP, Kemper WS, Ross J Jr: Dissociation between regional myocardial dysfunction and ECG changes during ischemia in the conscious dog. Circulation 62:735, 1980
6. Beaupre PN, Cahalan MK, Kremer PF et al: Does pulmonary artery occlusion pressure adequately reflect left ventricular filling during anesthesia and surgery? (abstr). Anesthesiology 59:A3, 1983
7. Roizen MF, Hunt TK, Beaupre PN et al: The effect of alpha-adrenergic

blockade on cardiac performance and tissue oxygen delivery during excision of pheochromocytoma. Surgery 94:941, 1983

8. Roizen MF, Beaupre PN, Alpert RA et al: Monitoring with two-dimensional transesophageal echocardiography. J Vasc Surg 1:300, 1984
9. Topol EJ, Weiss JL, Guzman PA et al: Immediate improvement of dysfunctional myocardial segments after coronary revascularization: Detection by intraoperative transesophageal echocardiography. J Am Coll Cardiol 4:1123, 1984
10. Smith JS, Cahalan MK, Benefiel DJ et al: Intraoperative detection of myocardial ischemia in high-risk patients: Electrocardiography versus two-dimensional transesophageal echocardiography. Circulation 72:1015, 1985
11. Konstadt SN, Thys D, Mindich BP, Kaplan JA, Goldman M: Validation of quantitative intraoperative transesophageal echocardiography. Anesthesiology 65:418, 1986
12. Shively B, Watters T, Benefiel D, Cahalan MK, Botvonick EH, Schiller NB: The intraoperative detection of myocardial infarction by transesophageal echocardiography (abstr). J Am Coll Cardiol 7:2A, 1986
13. Gewertz BL, Kremser PC, Zarins CK et al: Transesophageal echocardiographic monitoring of myocardial ischemia during vascular surgery. J Vasc Surg 5:607, 1987
14. Koolen JJ, Visser CA, van Wezel HB, Meyne NG, Dunning AJ: Influence of coronary artery bypass surgery on regional left ventricular wall motion: An intraoperative two-dimensional transesophageal echocardiographic study. J Cardiovasc Anes 1:273, 1987
15. Abel MD, Nishimura RA, Callahan MJ, Rehder K, Ilstrup DM, Tajik AJ: Evaluation of intraoperative transesophageal two-dimensional echocardiography. Anesthesiology 66:64, 1987
16. Slavik JR, LaMantia KR, Kopriva CJ, Prokop E, Ezekowitz MD, Barash PG: Does nitrous oxide cause regional wall motion abnormalities in patients with coronary artery disease? Anesth Analg 67:695, 1988
17. London MJ, Tubau JF, Wong MG, Layug E, Mangano DT: The "natural history" of segmental wall motion abnormalities detected by intraoperative transesophageal echocardiography: A clinically blinded, prospective approach (abstr). Anesthesiology 69:A7, 1988
18. O'Kelly BF, Knight AA, Tubau JF, Verrier ED, Mangano DT: Intraoperative measurement of left ventricular contractility (abstr). Circulation 74 (suppl):II-479, 1988
19. Smith JS, Roizen MF, Cahalan MK et al: Does anesthetic technique make a difference? Augmentation of systolic blood pressure during carotid endarterectomy: Effects of phenylephrine versus light anesthesia and of isoflurane versus halothane on the incidence of myocardial ischemia. Anesthesiology 69:846, 1988
20. Leung JM, O'Kelly BF, Browner WS, Tubau JF, Hollenberg M, Mangano DT: Prognostic importance of postbypass regional wall motion abnormalities in patients undergoing coronary artery bypass graft surgery. Anesthesiology 71:16, 1989
21. Saada M, Cahalan MK, Lee E, Schiller NB: Real-time evaluation of segmental wall motion abnormalities (abstr). Anesth Analg 68:S242, 1989
22. Leung JM, O'Kelly B, Helman J et al: Risk of myocardial ischemia during

sufentanil vs. isoflurane anesthesia as assessed by transesophageal echocardiography (abstr). Anesthesiology 71:A1164, 1989
23. Falsetti HL, Marcus ML, Kerber RE, Skorton DJ: Quantification of myocardial ischemia and infarction by left ventricular imaging. Circulation 63:747, 1981
24. Falsetti HL, Mates RE, Grant C, Greene DG, Bunnell IL: Left ventricular wall stress calculated from one-plane cineangiography. Circ Res 26:71, 1970
25. Vine DL, Hegg TD, Dodge HT, Stewart DK, Frimer M: Immediate effect of contrast medium injection on left ventricular volumes and ejection fraction: A study using metallic epicardial markers. Circulation 56:379, 1977
26. Carroll RJ, Verani MS, Falsetti HL: The effect of collateral circulation on segmental left ventricular contraction. Circulation 50:709, 1974
27. Schnittger I, Fitzgerald PJ, Gordon EP, Alderman AL, Popp RL: Computerized quantitative analysis of left ventricular wall motion by two-dimensional echocardiography. Circulation 70:242, 1984
28. Skorton DJ, Collins SM, Kerber RE: Digital processing and analysis in echocardiography. In Collins SM, Skorton DJ (eds): Cardiac Imaging and Image Processing, pp. 171–205. New York, McGraw-Hill, 1986
29. Force T, Bloomfield P, O'Boyle JE, Khuri SF, Josa M, Parisi AF: Quantitative two-dimensional echocardiographic analysis of regional wall motion in patients with perioperative myocardial infarction. Circulation 70:233, 1984
30. Durkin M, Lehmann KG, Kopriva CJ et al: 2D-transesophageal echocardiography: Are all regional wall motion abnormalities harbingers of myocardial ischemia? (abstr). Anesthesiology 63:A66, 1985
31. Leung JM, Chan FW, Mangano DT: Transesophageal echocardiography: Prediction of intraoperative hypovolemia (abstr). Anesth Analg 70:S236, 1990
32. Reichek N, Wilson J, St John Sutton M, Plappert TA, Goldberg S, Hirshfeld JW: Noninvasive determination of left ventricular end-systolic stress: Validation of the method and initial application. Circulation 65:99, 1982
33. St John Sutton MG, Plappert TA, Hirshfeld JW, Reichek N: Assessment of left ventricular mechanics in patients with asymptomatic aortic regurgitation: A two-dimensional echocardiographic study. Circulation 69:259, 1984
34. Quinones MA, Moketoff DM, Nouri S, Winters WL Jr, Miller RR: Noninvasive quantification of left ventricular wall stress. Am J Cardiol 45:782, 1980
35. Grossman W, Braunwald E, Mann T, McLaurin LP, Green LH: Contractile state of the left ventricle in man as evaluated from end-systolic pressure-volume relations. Circulation 56:845, 1977
36. Schluter M, Hinrich A, Thier W et al: Transesophageal two-dimensional echocardiography: Comparison of ultrasonic and anatomic sections. Am J Cardiol 53:1173, 1984
37. Heger JJ, Weyman AE, Wann LS, Dillon JC, Feigenbaum H: Cross-sectional echocardiography in acute myocardial infarction: Detection and localization of regional left ventricular asynergy. Circulation 60:531, 1979
38. Lieberman AN, Weiss JL, Jugdutt BI et al: Two-dimensional echocardiography and infarct size: Relationship of regional wall motion and thicken-

ing to the extent of myocardial infarction in the dog. Circulation 63:739, 1981
39. Lima JAC, Becker LC, Melin JA et al: Impaired thickening of nonischemic myocardium during acute regional ischemia in the dog. Circulation 71:1048, 1985
40. London MJ, Tubau JF, Harris D et al: Dipyridamole thallium imaging predicts intraoperative ischemia in patients undergoing major vascular surgery (abstr). J Am Coll Cardiol 11:162A, 1988
41. Watters TA, Dae MW, Botvinick EH et al: The relationship between myocardium at ischemic risks and induced intraoperative ischemia: Prognostic implications (abstr). J Am Coll Cardiol 11:186A, 1988

Thomas E. Stanley

5 Quantitative Echocardiography

Quantitative analysis of the physiologic information available in two-dimensional echocardiograms is a process that has been developed and validated for nearly as long as two-dimensional imaging technology has been available.[1] However, most cardiologists readily acknowledge that such numerical measurement techniques are seldom used in the routine implementation of precordial echocardiography. Two basic reasons exist for this fact. First, in most cases, a subjective, qualitative interpretation of cardiac performance has been adequate for the purposes for which a periodic bedside echocardiogram is obtained. Assessments that use echocardiography under these conditions might be considered analogous to establishing the patient's New York Heart Association (NYHA) classification for left ventricular function, in which the typical qualitative scoring system (Table 5-1) is used to confirm a clinical impression. The second reason for the limited use of quantitative methods in echocardiography is the fact that they are *tedious* processes that require a relatively large amount of time as well as diligent attention to detail and concentration by the operator.

The development of the transesophageal ultrasound transducer has allowed continuous cardiac imaging to enter the intraoperative environment. Transesophageal echocardiography (TEE) has several important advantages: high-quality images are obtainable because the esophageal approach has a relatively close and unobstructed view of

TABLE 5-1. Subjective Scoring of Cardiac Function in Echocardiography

Score	Meaning
Normal	No evidence of dysfunction
Mild hypokinesia	Minimal diminution in function
Moderate hypokinesia	Significantly abnormal movement or thickening
Severe hypokinesia	Barely perceptible movement
Akinesia	Total lack of movement or thickening
Dyskinesia	Paradoxical outward movement or wall thinning

the heart; stable, consistent imaging is available for prolonged periods without contamination of the surgical field. In this way, TEE provides a means of constantly monitoring cardiac function.

The requirements for echocardiography to become an intraoperative cardiac monitor are significantly different than those placed on this technology in other settings. Patients who are undergoing surgery can experience rapid changes in hemodynamics and cardiovascular status. These changes demand frequent functional assessments, as well as the ability to compare all of these measurements from the various times in the patient's course. As a parallel to the aforementioned analogy for intermittent precordial echocardiograms and NYHA class, the data from intraoperative TEE monitoring ideally should attain the more objective characteristics of serial cardiac output determinations.

Routine clinical use and interpretation of TEE information is dependent on the training of the operator to recognize and to subjectively "quantify" cardiac function. Changes in cardiac function during a case that might warrant an intervention, thus, are established solely from the abilities and the memory of the observer. Clements and colleagues established that anesthesiologists can be successfully trained to recognize new abnormalities in regional myocardial function in TEE images.[2] However, Hillel and coworkers reported less favorable results in the subjective estimation of left ventricular ejection fraction.[3] Also, Saada and associates found that echocardiographic episodes of dysfunction consistent with myocardial ischemia were frequently missed during real-time observations and subjective interpretations of the TEE.[4] Finally, a recent study by Lazar and colleagues demonstrated that qualitative scoring techniques failed to distinguish an improvement in regional myocardial function following coronary revascularization that a more precise, quantitative analysis of segmental wall thickening in the same echocardiographic images demonstrated.[5] Clearly, the importance of objective techniques of echocardiographic analysis is amplified by the advent of its intraoperative use with transesophageal imaging.

In this chapter, current methods of quantitation of two-dimensional echocardiographic information is reviewed. In addition, the use of contrast echocardiography as an indicator of myocardial perfusion is discussed from the standpoint of quantitative techniques.

ECHOCARDIOGRAPHIC IMAGING

To understand numerical measurements of echocardiographic information as well as the limitations of these techniques, it is important that one be familiar with the physical process of image generation.

Ultrasonic representation of an object is performed by a transducer, which consists of a series of piezoelectric crystals that transmit a beam of high-frequency sound in a single direction. Sound energy reflected from an object's surface returns after a delay that is proportional to its distance from the transducer and with an intensity that is related to the distinctness of the surface. However, instead of being reflected totally in this *specular* or mirrorlike fashion, the beam may be partially *scattered* if the surface is small or irregular. This possibility adds to the complexity and imprecision of the returning ultrasound signal and is responsible for "echo dropouts" and missing surface representations in the final image.

Two-dimensional images are formed by sweeping multiple, individual beams across 80 to 90 degrees of arc. The time needed for performing an entire sweep of the sector arc is sufficiently short, so that the resulting image is considered a still frame of a moving object. Image processing steps performed in the scan conversion of these multiple radial lines into a rectangular video display include smoothing and interpolation of missing points at locations distant from the transducer (Fig. 5-1). The overall representation of the image is highly dependent on these processing steps as well as other user-controlled variables, such as the individual gain settings, which can often distort the perceived size or position of an object.

The two-dimensional scan is repeated 30 to 60 times per second. The human eye and brain are quite adept at assimilating these rapidly generated images, which create the illusion of continuous motion. This temporal integration is largely responsible for the ease with which the human observer can recognize objects within the images, since object recognition is made more difficult when only a single frame is available. On the other hand, it is nearly impossible for the observer to rapidly

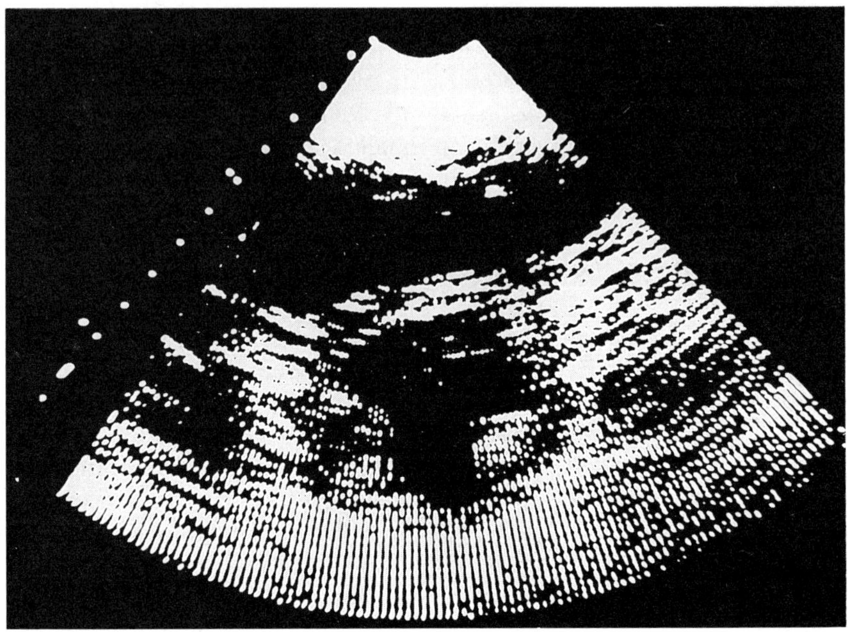

FIGURE 5-1. Two-dimensional echocardiographic image of the cardiac minor axis at the left ventricular midpapillary muscle level. Note in this rendering that the two-dimensional image is actually formed of multiple B mode scan lines and that, at locations distant to the transducer, these lines separate, leaving gaps in the image. Interpolation and smoothing techniques are used during scan conversion to create a more recognizable image. *(Koenigsberg DI, Ganote C: Anatomy of the heart as related to two-dimensional echocardiography. In: Talano JV. Cardiac Ultrasound Workbook, New York, Grune & Stratton, 1982.)*

TABLE 5-2. Basic Requirements in Quantitative Echocardiography

- Imaging performed during stable cardiac rhythm
  Example: Sinus, *not* postextrasystolic beat
- Reliable image of a *standard* two-dimensional view of the three-dimensional heart
  Example: Minor-axis midpapillary muscle view
- Description of the cardiac structure within the image
  Example: Recognition and circumferential outlining of the left ventricular endocardium
- Calculation of a physiologically meaningful parameter using the image description data
  Example: Area ejection fraction computation using end-diastolic and end-systolic images

perform any numerical analysis of the motion of these objects once they are identified. One must rely on the use of accessory computational tools that operate on the single frame images to complete the task of quantitative analysis.

Whatever purpose a particular quantitation scheme is designed to serve, several requirements are universal (Table 5-2). Analyses should be performed on images taken during a stable, consistent cardiac rhythm. A nonsinus beat or one that follows a premature contraction may not be representative of the otherwise ongoing cardiac functional profile of the patient. Secondly, a two-dimensional echocardiogram is only a single-plane representation of the three-dimensional structure of the heart. Thus, it is important that this two-dimensional view be a consistent anatomic "slice" of the heart. For instance, a number of planes might be considered to represent the minor-axis view of the left ven-

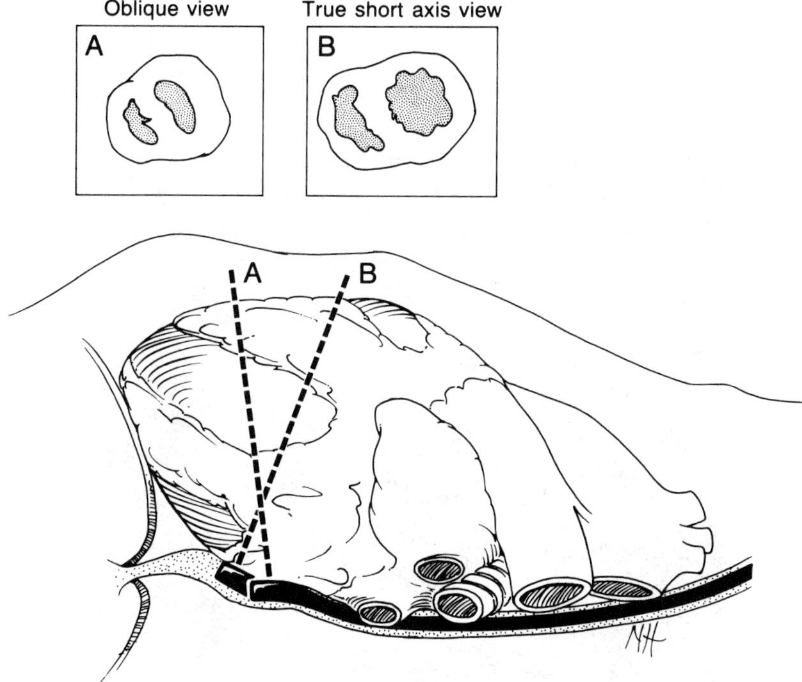

FIGURE 5-2. Diagrammatic view of thorax with the TEE probe positioned for a short- (minor) axis view of the ventricles. The image in plane *A* shows an oblique view, in which the ventricular walls appear falsely thick. The true short axis (plane *B*) is the preferable view and may require anterior flexion of the transducer element.

tricle (Fig. 5-2). However, only one minor-axis plane, a perpendicular slice at the midpapillary muscle level, is typically used for quantitative appraisal of global and regional left ventricular function.[5,6,7] Aberration from this plane results in the generation of widely variant numerical information.[8]

The next step in a quantitation process is to describe the cardiac structure of interest that is represented within the image. As an example, outlining of the endocardial border of the left ventricle in the minor-axis view is usually carried out by the operator using a tracing facility built into the echocardiograph machine (Fig. 5-3). This step requires that the objects be "recognized" from the available image data and is greatly facilitated by the use of *a priori* information of how the heart is known to appear in the selected projection. The human eye and brain are far more capable of this process than existing computerized image processors. Once described by this outlining, the anatomic information is available to the computer, which can execute the planned quantitation based on these data.

Finally, an appropriate, validated algorithm or mathematical process must be applied to the raw image description data to provide a

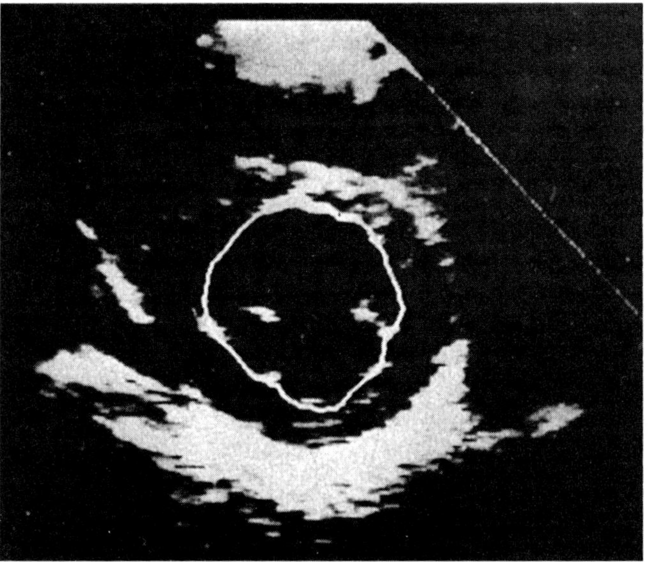

FIGURE 5-3. Echocardiographic minor-axis view of the left ventricle, with the endocardial surface outlined. The densities within the traced loop are the papillary muscles.

physiologically meaningful value. For instance, a computation of the area encompassed by the endocardial border of the left ventricle at both end-diastole and end-systole can be used to derive an area ejection fraction term that can help describe the patient's overall cardiac function.

QUANTITATION OF GLOBAL CARDIAC FUNCTION

Frequent assessment of overall cardiac performance has become an important facet of cardiovascular monitoring during anesthesia and in the critical care environment. An accepted standard for this form of monitoring is the measurement of cardiac output using the thermodilution technique. Another valuable measure of cardiovascular efficiency is the determination of left ventricular ejection fraction (LVEF), which is the difference between end-diastolic and end-systolic volumes (V_{ED}, V_{ES}, respectively) expressed as a percentage of V_{ED} (Equation 5-1).

$$\text{LVEF} = \frac{V_{ED} - V_{ES}}{V_{ED}} \cdot 100\% \qquad (5\text{-}1)$$

This measurement has been shown to be a predictor of outcome in studies that compare treatment modalities in patients with cardiac disease,[9,10] and, when available preoperatively, it is valuable to the anesthesiologist in planning care of these patients that present for surgery.

Determination of LVEF is made using radionuclide angiography, cineangiography, or echocardiography. Of these, only radionuclide studies measure actual volume of the ventricular cavity. Cineangiography and echocardiography are restricted to providing two-dimensional projections of the heart and, thus, display changes in left ventricular cavity area during the cardiac cycle. These data can be converted to an actual volume measurement using one of several algorithms (Fig. 5-4). While reasonable precision of left ventricular volume determination is possible with these formulas,[1,11] they are rather complex to implement within the fast-paced intraoperative environment, especially since many require information from multiple planes. A new, biplane transesophageal transducer may assist in the accuracy of these calculations by providing synchronous views of perpendicular image planes. Other investigations have shown that reasonable volume estimates may be made from single image data.[12] Thys and associates demonstrated a reasonable association between changes in left ventricular stroke volume computed from one minor-axis plane and cardiac output using thermodilution.[13] Clements and coworkers performed simulta-

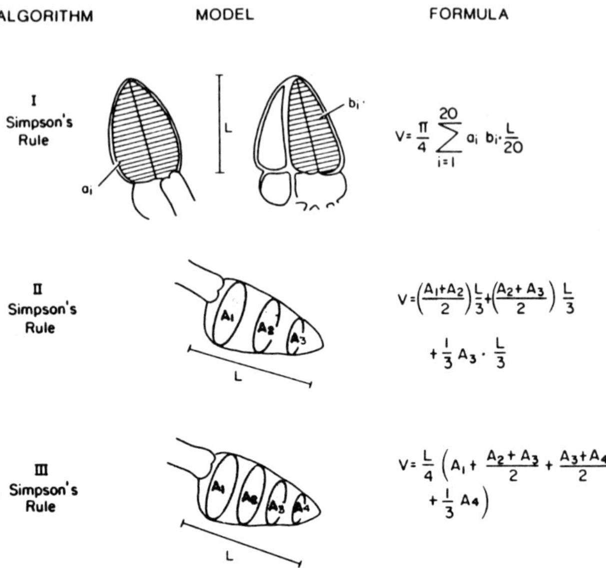

FIGURE 5-4. Biplane and single plane algorithms to calculate chamber volume from two-dimensional echocardiograms. *I,* Simpson's rule method based on orthogonal planes from the apical two-chamber and apical four-chamber planes. The calculation is based on the summation of areas from diameters ai and bi of 20 equal cylinders or discs. *II,III,* Simpson's rule using a summation of parasternal short-axis planes obtained from the apex to the base. *(continued)*

neous two-dimensional TEE and first-pass radionuclide angiograms (RNA) on patients who were undergoing major vascular surgery.[14] They reported that the TEE-derived minor-axis area ejection fraction alone provided a reasonable prediction of true volume ejection fraction as determined by RNA ($r = 0.96$).

The accuracy of the results of any of these analysis schemes can be affected significantly by other independent factors. Tracing of the endocardial outline is prone to error in recognizing which portion of the returned ultrasound signal is actually that boundary. Although the true two-dimensional endocardial edge is a discrete, vanishingly small ring, echocardiographic imaging gives this border a finite degree of thickness. The gain settings of the instrument significantly affect this thickness, with higher gains resulting in a "thicker" boundary. Thus, a border has

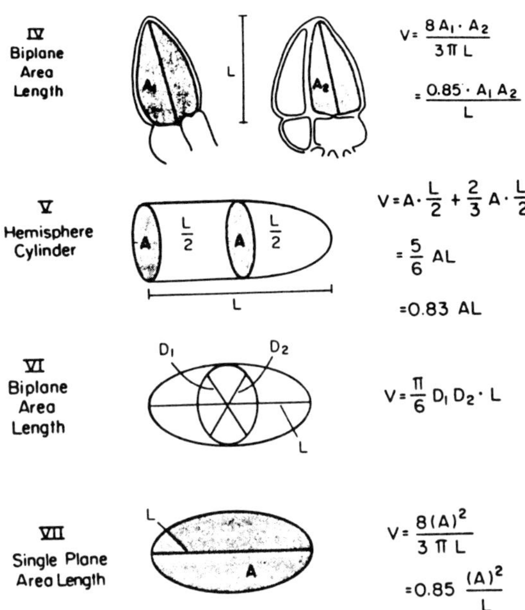

FIGURE 5-4. (*continued*) *IV,* Biplane area-length method of the traced area outlines (A1 and A2) obtained from the apical two-chamber and four-chamber planes. *V,* The hemispheric cylinder model uses an area obtained from the parasternal short axis plane and a length from an apical plane. *VI,* Ellipsoid plane technique using the length obtained from an apical plane. *VII,* Single plane area length method. *(Adapted from Silverman NH, Snider AR: Two-dimensional Echocardiography in Congenital Heart Disease. Norwalk, Appleton-Century-Crofts, 1982)*

a leading and trailing edge (closer to and farther from the transducer, respectively). This is especially apparent in the portions of the edge that are perpendicular to the ultrasound beam (Fig. 5-5). Tracing the area of the endocardial cavity, for example, makes it possible to identify the boundaries of the endocardium by using any permutation of the two leading and trailing edges. However, depending on the amount of thickness given to the boundaries, a trailing edge–leading edge analysis produces different results from a leading edge–trailing edge technique. Wyatt and colleagues studied the influence of these variations on the

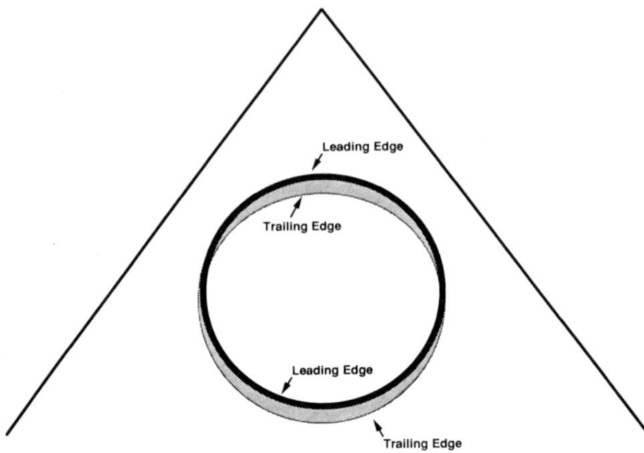

FIGURE 5-5. Stylized diagram of an echocardiogram imaging a circular structure, such as the endocardial surface of the left ventricle in the minor-axis view. The gray area indicates the "thickness" of this surface, which is most prevalent at the points where the ultrasound beam is perpendicular to the surface. Thus, two leading edge–trailing edge combinations are present. The black trace indicates a leading edge–leading edge outline of the surface, which yields the most accurate results.

accuracy of linear and area measurements of echocardiograms and reported that only the leading edge–leading edge method resulted in acceptable correlations to direct in vitro observations.[15]

Clearly, hemodynamic indices, such as heart rate, preload, and afterload, play major roles in determining the cardiac function. It is especially important that these factors be borne in mind and either controlled or accounted for when quantitative echocardiography is used in research to measure the effect of a separate intervention.

QUANTITATION OF REGIONAL CARDIAC FUNCTION

While knowledge of the global function of the left ventricle is a useful facet of cardiac monitoring, the ability of echocardiography to describe the contributions of individual regions of the myocardium to overall cardiac function sets it apart from all other monitoring systems. Myocardial ischemia is, in general, a regional phenomenon, with diminished blood flow to various areas of tissue determined by the presence and severity of obstructions in the various coronary arteries. It has been known since 1935 that the contractile function of the heart is sensitive to the adequacy of its perfusion. Tennant and Wiggers published what has become a classic work that demonstrates an immediate decrease in the force of contraction in hearts after occlusion of a coronary artery.[16] Thus, detection of regional cardiac dysfunction in response to acute ischemia constitutes an important role for echocardiography in the intraoperative setting. This need is emphasized by the concept that intraoperative myocardial ischemia may lead to postoperative myocardial infarction.[17]

Quantitation of regional left ventricular function has been implemented by measuring the change in motion of various segments of the endocardium between diastole and systole. Either the major- or minor-axis may be used for this analysis (Fig. 5-6). An outline of the endocardial border at end-systole is superimposed on a similar trace at end-diastole. A number of chords or radii are constructed, usually from a

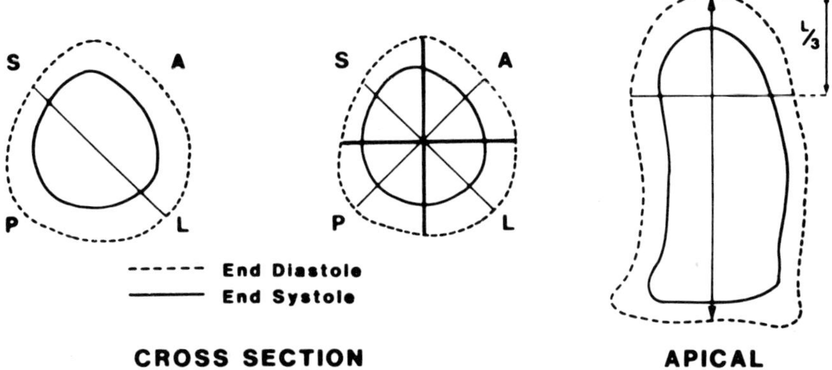

FIGURE 5-6. Conventions used for different degrees of subdivision of short-axis images. *Left,* An initial septolateral *(S,L)* axis, constructed to divide the diastolic and overlaid systolic outlines into anterior *(A)* and posterior *(P)* halves. *Center,* Further subdivision of the left ventricle outlined into octants is demonstrated. The four bolder hemiaxes indicate the regions used for the quadrant analysis. *Right,* The approach for defining the apical region of contraction from the outlines of the apical, long-axis view. *(Adapted from Moynihan PF, Parisi AF, Feldman CL: Quantitative detection of regional left ventricular contraction abnormalities by two-dimensional echocardiography. I. Analysis of methods. Circulation 63:752, 1981)*

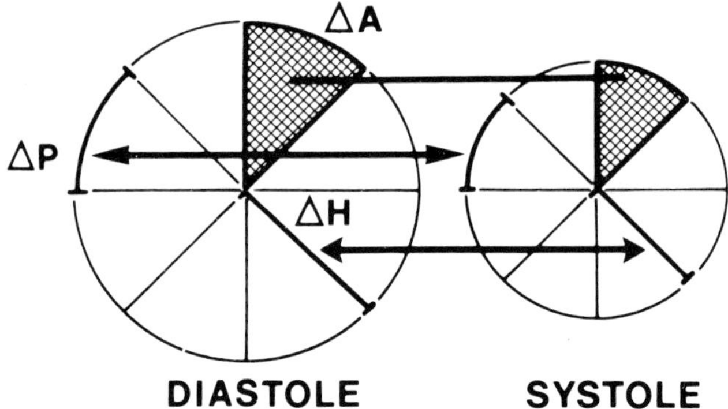

FIGURE 5-7. Schematic of diastolic and systolic left ventricular outlines subdivided into octants showing different approaches to measuring regional contraction. **Δ*A*,** regional area change; **Δ*H*,** hemiaxis shortening; **Δ*P*,** segmental endocardial perimeter contraction. *(Adapted from Moynihan PF, Parisi AF, Feldman CL: Quantitative detection of regional left ventricular contraction abnormalities by two-dimensional echocardiography. I. Analysis of methods. Circulation 63:752, 1981)*

central point of the outlines, to determine the motion of individual regions of the left ventricular circumference. This motion can be expressed as a change in axis length, circumferential shortening, or regional area (Fig. 5-7). Schnittger and associates studied these techniques in patients with both normal and abnormal cardiac function and found no significant differences in sensitivity, specificity, or reproducibility between area and length methods of determining segmental left ventricular function,[18] while other investigators found a slight advantage in using the segmental area change method.[19,20]

When the endocardial border is divided into segments to specify regional function, assignment or referencing between sequential cardiac images must be established so that comparisons can identify the same segments of myocardium. In addition to contracting, the heart rotates and shifts (translates) in the thorax between diastole and systole. Failure to correct for these motion artifacts may result in a misleading analysis of cardiac contraction. However, when only the motion of the endocardial outline is examined, such correction is difficult to perform.[21] An example of this problem is seen in the use of the "floating" axis system, which aligns end-diastolic and end-systolic images by superimposing their computed "centers of mass" (Fig. 5-8). A dyskinetic

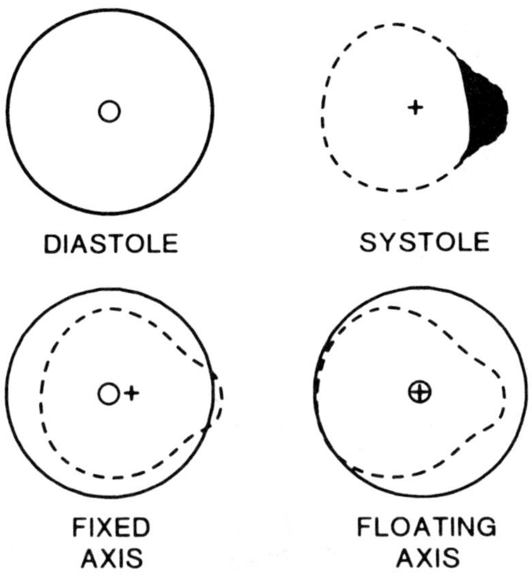

FIGURE 5-8. Demonstration of the shortcomings of endocardial wall motion referencing systems in evaluating regional cardiac contraction. *Upper panels,* End-diastolic *(solid contour)* and end-systolic *(dotted contour)* are shown for a cardiac cycle in which dyskinesia *(shaded bulge)* has occurred. *Lower panels,* The fixed-axis method *(left)* allows recognition of this dyskinetic segment but cannot identify true translational or rotational artifact. The floating-axis system *(right)* superimposes the centers of each image, an act which may cause the dyskinetic area to appear more normal and the normal wall to appear hypokinetic or akinetic. *(Skorton DJ, Collins SM, Kerber RE: Digital processing and analysis in echocardiography. In Collins SM, Skorton DJ (eds): Cardiac Imaging and Image Processing. New York, McGraw-Hill, 1986)*

bulge at end-systole results in a shift of the computed center toward the abnormal segment. Alignment of the centers of the two images, supposedly to correct for a translational artifact, in fact falsely minimizes the amount of dyskinesia actually present. Using a "fixed" axis system avoids this kind of error but does not account for translational or rotational movement when it truly occurs.

Measurement of systolic wall thickening is a means to avoid many such analysis errors. By encompassing the epicardial outline in the quantitation process, an act which causes the measurement chords to overlie the entire mass of the myocardium, much of the overall cardiac motion artifact can be corrected without losing sight of physiologic motion changes. In addition, a system for orienting thickness vectors along a "center-line" axis has been adapted for this purpose by Stanley

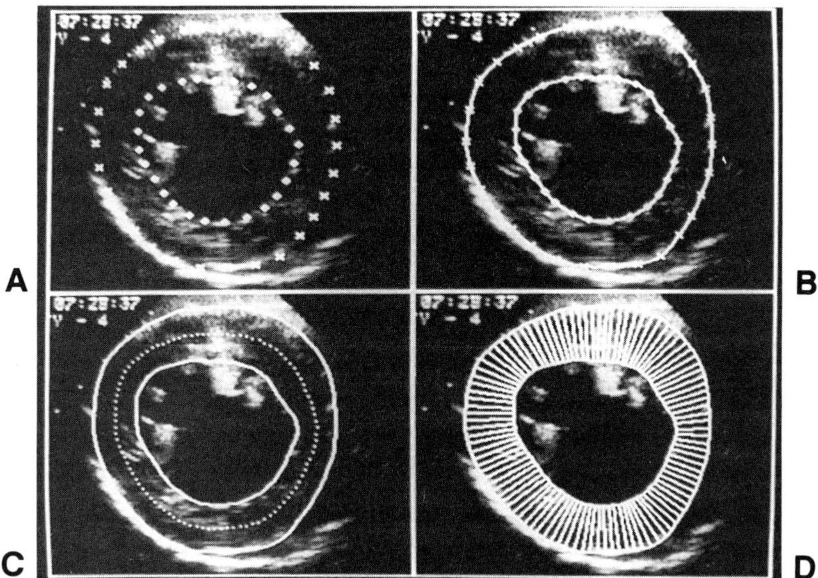

FIGURE 5-9. Steps in center line wall thickness determination. *A,* Endocardial and epicardial points are chosen around the circumference of a minor-axis image. *B,* Remaining points of outlines are interpolated using a cubic polynomial algorithm. *C,* A set of 100 points equidistant from the two outlines is computed as a center line. *D,* Wall thickness chords are constructed as perpendiculars to tangents around the center line and intersect the original outlines. *(Stanley TE III, Skelton TN, de Bruijn NP: Centerline systolic wall thickening: A method for quantitating regional cardiac function using transesophageal echocardiography. Anesth Analg 68:S275, 1989)*

and colleagues[22] from the work of Sheehan and associates, who devised this method to track endocardial motion from ventricular cineangiograms.[23] An advantage of the center-line technique is that the thickness chords are relatively independent vectors and better represent the regional thickness measurement than if a single reference point were chosen and the chords drawn radically (Fig. 5-9). Also, the numbering of chords around the circumference of the minor axis can be oriented to a fixed anatomic structure, such as a papillary muscle, resulting in correction of rotational artifact.

Systolic wall thickening may be a more accurate descriptor of ischemic changes than simple endocardial wall motion. Ren and associates described systolic wall thickening abnormalities in 92% to 100% of patients who had ventricular dysfunction documented by angiography.[24] Endocardial wall motion abnormalities were present in only 46% to 60% of these patients. Gallagher and colleagues demonstrated significant decreases in systolic wall thickening with progressive reductions in coronary blood flow.[25] Laboratory and clinical studies have shown excellent correlation of echocardiographically measured systolic wall thickening changes with the onset of myocardial ischemia.[26,27]

QUANTITATION OF CONTRAST ECHOCARDIOGRAPHY

The extreme difference in acoustic impedance between air and blood causes air bubbles to be strongly reflective of ultrasound. Exceptionally small bubbles (2–100 μm) can be visualized by echocardiography, making this technique a most sensitive means of diagnosing air bubbles in the circulation.

This reflectivity of air bubbles can be put to use safely as a "contrast agent" in echocardiography, provided that the bubbles are of sufficiently small size. By vigorously agitating saline or another injectable vehicle, cavitation and mixing with surrounding air cause the formation of microbubbles. The microbubbles created by hand agitation are slightly larger than red blood cells (about 15 μm diameter) but have a short half-life in the circulation (2–3 minutes).

Direct coronary artery injection of microbubble solutions during cardiac catheterization[28] and coronary artery bypass surgery[29] has provided ultrasonic visualization of regional myocardial perfusion. This technique requires more carefully prepared microbubbles, usually using sonicated Renografin solution, which provides a smaller bubble diameter (5 μm) and has been used safely in cardiac surgical patients.[30] Echo-

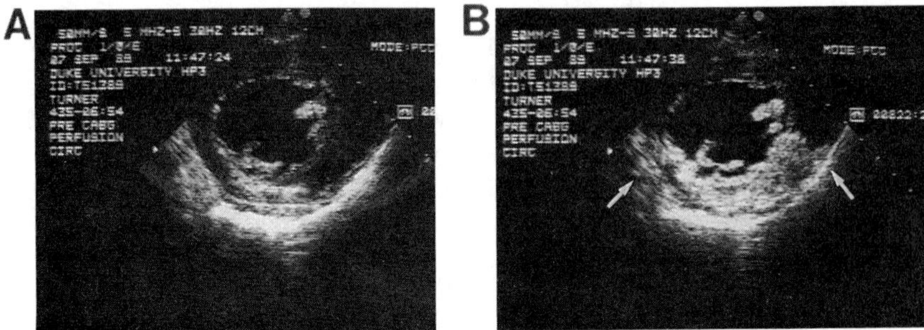

FIGURE 5-10. Epicardial short-axis echocardiograph of the left ventricle at the midpapillary muscle level *(anterior structures at the top). A,* During cardiopulmonary bypass immediately prior to contrast injection into a saphenous vein graft to the second and third circumflex marginal coronary arteries. *B,* Same view at peak contrast intensity after the injection of 2 ml of sonicated Renografin directly into the bypass graft. Perfusion of the entire posterior left ventricle, the posterior septum, and both papillary muscles is clearly visualized *(area between the white arrows).* *(Smith PK, Stanley TE III: Intraoperative contrast echocardiography: A direct approach to measure regional myocardial perfusion. Anesthesiology 72:219, 1990)*

cardiographic imaging during coronary artery injection of these microbubbles results in a transient increase in reflected ultrasound signal in the regions of myocardium that are perfused by that coronary vascular bed (Fig. 5-10). The intensity and time course of this contrast enhancement is in proportion to blood flow in the coronary artery.

Aronson and coworkers demonstrated in an animal model that the appearance of myocardial contrast enhancement reliably predicted patency or experimental occlusion of a coronary artery ($p < .01$).[31] This association was determined using a subjective assessment of the echocardiograms by the investigators for the presence or absence of contrast enhancement. Clearly, a more objective, better-quantitated approach is necessary for widespread use of this technique. Computerized image processing provides a great deal of flexibility in performing such analyses, allowing digital "subtraction" of irrelevant background information, as well as numerical interpretation of contrast by assignment to a "gray level" value. If serial images taken during a microbubble injection are measured in this way, contrast intensity can be plotted against time, providing a reflection of blood flow (Fig. 5-11). Vandenberg and associates studied contrast echocardiography using computerized processing and found a fair correlation between experimental changes in cor-

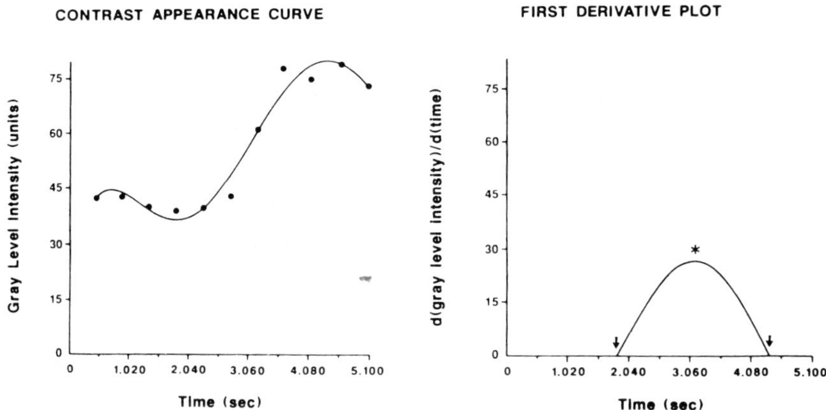

FIGURE 5-11. *Left,* Gray level intensity data vs. time are fitted to a fifth-order polynomial regression model. ***Right,*** A first derivative of the polynomial regression model provides the determination of the maximal slope of the appearance curve *(*)* and time from baseline to peak contrast appearance ***(between arrows).*** *(Vandenberg BF, Kieso R, Fox-Eastham K et al: Quantitation of myocardial perfusion by contrast echocardiography: Analysis of contrast grey level appearance variables and intracyclic variability. J Am Coll Cardiol 13:200, 1989)*

onary artery blood flow and changes in maximal slope of the contrast appearance curve (r = .77).[32] Time to occurrence of the contrast peak bore no relation to blood flow (r = .14).

Many obstacles remain in the development of quantitative contrast echocardiography. The most commonly used contrast vehicle, sonicated Renografin solution, creates microbubbles that are excessively variable in size. Since reflection and scattering of ultrasound is not linearly related to bubble diameter, it becomes difficult to model the intensity of returned signal to predict precisely the amount or appearance rate of the vehicle and, therefore, the blood flow. The advent of contrast agents with more uniform reflective surfaces, such as air-encasing albumin or polysaccharide microspheres, will simplify this task.

FUTURE ENHANCEMENTS IN QUANTITATIVE ECHOCARDIOGRAPHY

A serious impediment to the routine use of any available quantitative analysis scheme in echocardiography is the requirement for a significant amount of user interaction. The operator must trace cardiac outlines on a frozen video image to make measurements. This process consumes too much time to be a practical part of intraoperative monitoring with TEE.

Computer analysis and image processing in echocardiography is a well-established field of research, and on-line automatic computerized image recognition and processing is the ultimate goal that will solve this problem.[21] However, progress in this area has been restrained by poor signal-to-noise ratios in the echocardiographic image, as well as the lack of a mathematically clear, comprehensive understanding of the interaction of ultrasound with biologic tissue. Improvements in overall image quality by enhanced TEE technology and the development of powerful, portable computer resources may finally allow implementation of the complex algorithms that will be needed to objectively replicate what the observer's eye and brain subjectively perform. Porembka and colleagues recently reported successes with near real-time automated detection and display of the endocardial outline of the left ventricle from minor-axis echocardiograms.[33] Processing time was a scant 8 seconds per image and was successful with 80% to 95% of the images subjected to the analysis. Moreover, correlation of the computer-determined outline to those later drawn manually was excellent (r = .98).

The final implementation of systems such as these requires the interest and cooperation of echocardiograph manufacturers, since direct incorporation of the analysis technology with the image capture and display electronics will be the only practical means to provide these tools for general use.

References

1. Schiller NB, Drew D, Acquatella H et al: Noninvasive biplane quantitation of left ventricular volume and ejection fraction with real-time two-dimensional echocardiography system. Circulation 54(suppl):234, 1976
2. Clements FM, Hill R, Kisslo J et al: How easily can we learn to recognize regional wall motion abnormalities with 2D-transesophageal echocardiography (abstr). Anesthesiology 65:A478, 1986
3. Hillel Z, Thys D, Ali J: Can left ventricular ejection fraction be estimated by visual inspection of 2D-echocardiographic images? Proceedings of the Society of Cardiovascular Anesthesiologists, 11th Annual Meeting, Seattle, 1989
4. Saada M, Cahalan MK, Lee E et al: Real-time evaluation of segmental wall-motion abnormalities (abstr). Anesth Analg 68:S242, 1989
5. Lazar HL, Plehn J, Schick EM et al: Effects of coronary revascularization on regional wall motion. J Thorac Cardiovasc Surg 98:498, 1989

6. Leung JM, O'Kelly B, Browner WS et al: Prognostic importance of post-bypass regional wall-motion abnormalities in patients undergoing coronary artery bypass graft surgery. Anesthesiology 71:16, 1989
7. Topol EJ, Weiss JL, Guzman PA et al: Immediate improvement of dysfunctional myocardial segments after coronary revascularization: Detection by intraoperative transesophageal echocardiography. J Am Coll Cardiol 4:1123, 1984
8. Haendchen RV, Wyatt HL, Maurer G et al: Quantitation of regional cardiac function by two-dimensional echocardiography. I. Patterns of contraction of the normal left ventricle. Circulation 67:1234, 1983
9. Pryor DB, Harrell FE, Rankin JS et al: The changing survival benefits of coronary revascularization over time. Circulation 76:V13, 1987
10. Parisi AF, Khuri S, Deupree RH et al: Medical compared with surgical management of unstable angina: 5-year mortality and morbidity in the Veterans Administration Study. Circulation 80(suppl):I151, 1989
11. Folland ED, Parisi AF, Moynihan PF et al: Assessment of left ventricular ejection fraction and volumes by real-time, two dimensional echocardiography. Circulation 60:760, 1979
12. Parisi AF, Moynihan PF, Feldman CL et al: Approaches to the determination of left ventricular volume and ejection fraction by real-time two dimensional echocardiography. Clin Cardiol 2:257, 1979
13. Thys DM, Hillel Z, Goldman M et al: A comparison of hemodynamic indices derived by invasive monitoring and by two-dimensional echocardiography. Anesthesiology 65:A143, 1986
14. Clements FM, Harpole D, Quill TJ et al: Simultaneous measurement of cardiac volumes, areas and ejection fractions by transesophageal echocardiography and first pass radionuclide angiography (abstr). Anesthesiology 69:A4, 1988
15. Wyatt HL, Haendchen RV, Meerbaum S et al: Assessment of quantitative methods for 2-dimensional echocardiography. Am J Cardiol 52:396, 1983
16. Tennant R, Wiggers CJ: Effects of coronary occlusion on myocardial contraction. Am J Physiol 112:351, 1935
17. Slogoff S, Keats AS: Does perioperative myocardial ischemia lead to postoperative myocardial infarction? Anesthesiology 62:107, 1985
18. Schnittger I, Fitzgerald PJ, Gordon EP et al: Computerized quantitative analysis of left ventricular wall motion by two-dimensional echocardiography. Circulation 70:242, 1984
19. Grube E, Hanisch JL, Neumann J et al: Quantitative evaluation of LV-wall motion by two-dimensional echocardiography (2-DE) (abstr). J Am Coll Cardiol 1:581, 1983
20. Parisi AF, Moynihan PF, Folland ED et al: Quantitative detection of regional left ventricular contraction abnormalities by two-dimensional echocardiography. II. Accuracy in coronary artery disease. Circulation 63:761, 1981
21. Skorton DJ, Collins SM, Kerber RE: Digital image processing and analysis in echocardiography. In Collins SM, Skorton DJ (eds): Cardiac Imaging and Image Processing, pp. 171–205. New York, McGraw-Hill, 1986
22. Stanley TE III, Skelton TN, de Bruijn NP: Centerline systolic wall thickening: A method for quantitating regional cardiac function using transesophageal echocardiography (abstr). Anesth Analg 68:S275, 1989

23. Sheehan FH, Bolson EL, Dodge HT et al: Advantages and applications of the centerline method for characterizing regional ventricular function. Circulation 74:293, 1986
24. Ren JF, Kotler M, Hakki A et al: Quantitation of regional left ventricular function by two-dimensional echocardiography in normals and patients with coronary artery disease. Am Heart J 110:552, 1985
25. Gallagher KP, Kumada T, Koziol JA et al: Significance of regional wall thickening abnormalities relative to transmural myocardial perfusion in anesthetized dogs. Circulation 62:1266, 1980
26. Pandian NG, Kerber RE: Two-dimensional echocardiography in experimental coronary stenosis. I. Sensitivity and specificity in detecting transient myocardial dyskinesis: Comparison with sonomicrometers. Circulation 66:597, 1982
27. Kerber RE, Taylor AL, Hiratzka LF et al: Transient myocardial ischemia: Experimental echocardiographic demonstration and evaluation of myocardial contraction abnormalities. Can J Cardiol (suppl):136A, 1986
28. Cheirif J, Zoghbi WA, Raizner AE et al: Assessment of myocardial perfusion in humans by contrast echocardiography. I. Evaluation of regional coronary reserve by peak contrast intensity. J Am Coll Cardiol 11:735, 1988
29. Goldman ME, Mindich BP: Intraoperative cardioplegic contrast echocardiography for assessing myocardial perfusion during open heart surgery. J Am Coll Cardiol 4:1029, 1984
30. Kabas JS, Kisslo J, Flick CL et al: Intraoperative perfusion contrast echocardiography: A method to evaluate the effectiveness of coronary artery bypass grafting. J Thorac Cardiovasc Surg 99:536, 1990
31. Aronson S, Bender E, Feinstein SB et al: Contrast echocardiography: A method to visualize changes in regional myocardial perfusion in the dog model of CABG surgery. Anesthesiology 72:291, 1990
32. Vandenberg BF, Kieso R, Fox-Eastham K et al: Quantitation of myocardial perfusion by contrast echocardiography: Analysis of contrast grey level appearance variables and intracyclic variability. J Am Coll Cardiol 13:200, 1989
33. Porembka DT, Mintz R, Lin K et al: Automated on-line subcardial imagery of the mid-papillary region with transesophageal echocardiography (abstr). Anesthesiology 71:A343, 1989

Khalid H. Sheikh
David B. Adams
Joseph A. Kisslo

6 Doppler Color-Flow Imaging

Doppler color-flow imaging is a method for imaging blood flow through the heart by displaying flow data on the two-dimensional echocardiographic image. This ability has generated great excitement about the use of this method for identifying valvular, congenital, and other forms of heart disease as the color-flow image imparts spatial information to the Doppler data. Application of Doppler color-flow imaging in the operating room is especially exciting as it affords the unique opportunity to assess cardiac flows immediately before and after surgery, at a time when such information can be acted on. As the limitations in image quality imposed by the chest wall and lungs in conventional chest echocardiography are not a problem for two-dimensional or Doppler imaging when performed from either epicardial or transesophageal approaches, the quality of information is invariably excellent. What may ultimately be the most important factor in the introduction of echocardiography into the operating room is that, to inexperienced Doppler users, the color-flow display makes the Doppler data more readily understandable than conventional spectral Doppler modes. Thus, data that are more understandable are more likely to be used.

BASIC CONSIDERATIONS

An understanding of Doppler color-flow imaging requires an appreciation of Doppler principles, which are covered in Chapters 2 and 10. Using the frequency shift of ultrasound reflected from moving red blood cells, the direction, velocity, and character of blood flow can be determined. Normal blood flow is laminar, so that all of the red blood cells in a column of blood move in the same direction, with nearly the same velocity (Fig. 6-1A).[1] Disordered blood flow, as occurs in stenotic lesions, valvular regurgitation, and intracardiac shunts, is usually turbulent and has Doppler characteristics of multivelocity, multidirectional flow (Fig. 6-1B).

In contrast to spectral displays of blood-flow velocity, direction, and character, as are seen in both pulsed-wave and continuous-wave Doppler modes, Doppler color-flow imaging encodes the colors of red and blue to represent the direction of blood flow, and the various hues,

A

Laminar Flow

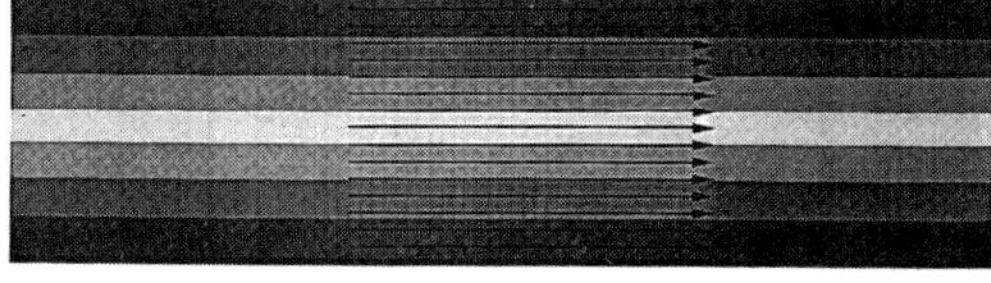

B

Turbulent Flow

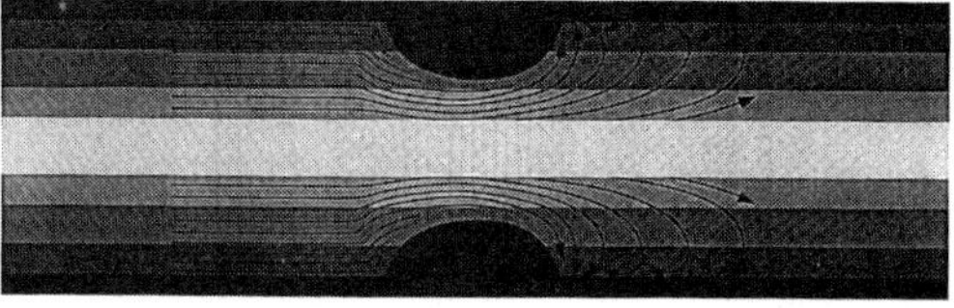

FIGURE 6-1. *A,* Laminar flow. All of the red blood cells are moving at approximately the same velocity and direction. *B,* Turbulent flow. The red blood cells have many different velocities and directions. *(After materials from the Irex corporation.)*

from dull to bright, represent the differing velocities. When turbulence is present, a mosaic of many colors results. A two-dimensional display of flow is, therefore, produced with ready identification of size, direction, velocity, and character of blood flow, which has spatial and temporal orientation relative to cardiac structures and events.

CREATION OF THE COLOR IMAGE

Reflected ultrasound data from any conventional scanner contains frequency shift information that results from the encounter of the transmitted ultrasound with moving structures and blood. Until the advent of color-flow imaging, these frequency shift data were simply ignored. Color-flow mapping uses the frequency shift data to assess red blood cell movement. Thus, color-flow imaging systems take advantage of data that are available in every ultrasound image of the heart.

Basics of Doppler Color-Flow Imaging

Doppler color-flow instruments are all based on pulsed Doppler methods. Conventional pulsed-wave techniques are range-gated, which means that, by knowing the speed of ultrasound in tissue, the Doppler

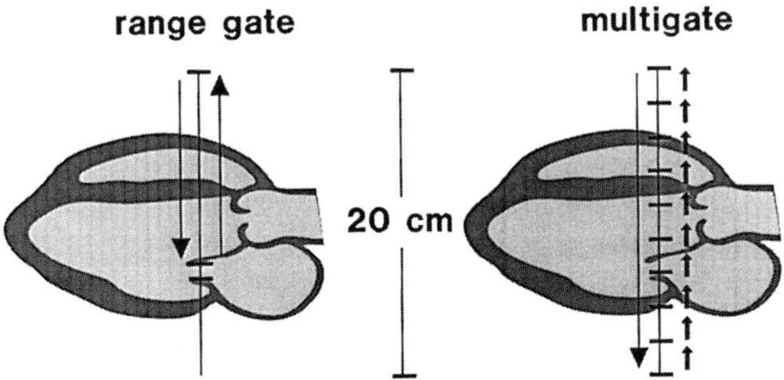

FIGURE 6-2. Color-flow Doppler systems use pulsed-wave Doppler principles in a multigate, rather than range-gate, format. *Left,* a conventional range-gated pulsed-wave Doppler system. *Right,* a multigated system where data are received from successive gates in range.

sample volume is determined in range by the time is takes for the ultrasound pulse to travel to the area of interest and then back. To encode velocities in color over a large area, without markedly compromising temporal resolution, color-flow systems are "multigated." In Figure 6-2, a conventional single-gate pulsed-wave approach is illustrated in the left-hand panel and compared with the simple ten-gate system in the right-hand panel. In the multigated format, a burst of ultrasound is sent into the tissue along a given line, and then the system rapidly receives data at 10 incremental times. This method permits sampling of multiple sites of flow in a short period of time.

Multigating takes advantage of Doppler information all along the line that is "ignored" in the conventional range-gated approach. It is good to think of the color-flow map image as comprised of little gates

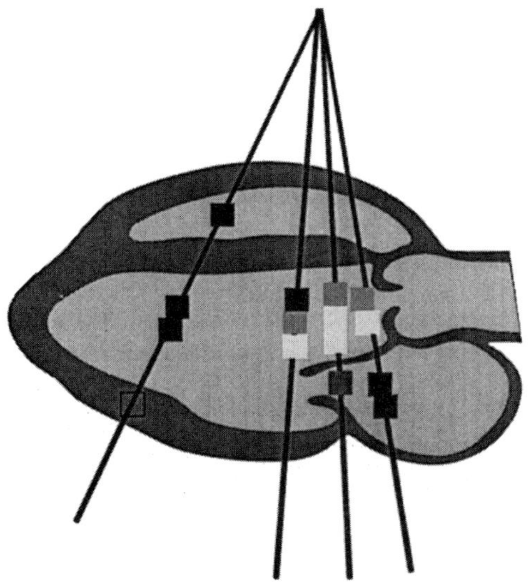

FIGURE 6-3. Hundreds of gates are present along each line everywhere in the color-flow image. In gates where there is target information, no color is displayed *(open gate at lower left).* In the final image, thousands of gates comprise each frame of the color image. Considerable time is required for calculation of phase shift information for each frame.

throughout the field of view, each gate containing some composite of the Doppler information. In reality, a typical image may be comprised of as many as 256 lines, depending on sector size and depth of range, with each line containing hundreds of gates (Fig. 6-3).

Color Display

All color systems are digitally based, which means that the complex flow data are assigned a number. In some ways, the creation of the color image may be likened to an electronic "paint by number" landscape. The key to color flow is to understand how the color system determines the number to be painted in each area. By convention, Doppler color-flow systems assign a given color to the direction of flow; red is flow toward and blue is flow away from the transducer. No flow is represented by black. Color reference bars always appear on the screen of Doppler flow imaging devices as a guide to the color encoding system that is in operation. Red blood cell mean velocity is displayed by the

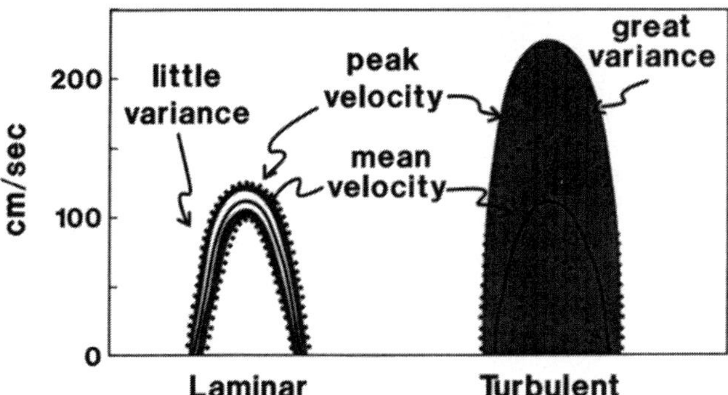

FIGURE 6-4. Schematic representation of a spectral recording showing the differences between peak and mean velocities. In the case of normal *laminar flow,* peak and mean velocities may be close. For *turbulent flow,* a significant difference may be found between peak and mean velocity. In *laminar flow,* little variation *(variance)* of velocities on either side of the mean velocity is seen. In *turbulent flow,* when many different velocities are present, great variance is seen.

color presented at each gate. Progressively increasing velocities are encoded in varying hues of either red or blue. The more dull the hue, the slower the velocity. The brighter the hue, the faster the relative velocity.

As shown in Figure 6-4, for normal laminar flow, mean and peak velocity are very close; whereas, in turbulent flow, velocities differ greatly, so that mean velocity may be only half of the peak velocity. Color maps which contain "variance" information take advantage of the discrepancies between mean and peak velocities to increase the available hues and colors available for display; in general, they make it easier to discriminate between normal and abnormal flow states.

Limitations and Technical Considerations

The technical requirements of Doppler color-flow imaging stress an ultrasound system that is already working to near maximum capacity in generating a two-dimensional image. Therefore, simultaneous two-dimensional and Doppler color-flow imaging require the use of separate image processors for each mode to generate a real-time image of simultaneous structure and flow. Even with a dedicated image processor, the generation of the Doppler color-flow image is a compromise among the factors that affect image quality and integrity. Among the factors directly under the control of the operator are transducer frequency, transducer orientation, and scan width and depth.

While a transducer orientation parallel to blood flow is critical for conventional pulsed-and continuous-wave Doppler assessment of peak flow velocity, it is not as crucial for color-flow imaging. Abnormal flow jets contain eddy currents that move in all directions. The color-flow exam is designed to recognize abnormal flows and not necessarily to characterize the peak velocity of the flow. However, once the abnormal flow is recognized, transducer manipulation is requried to completely define the size of the abnormal flow jet.

The accuracy of velocity measurements is directly related to the number of times flow at a given site is sampled. More time dedicated to sample flow at a particular site results in a better estimate of flow velocity at that site. However, too much sampling time results in a reduction in temporal resolution or a reduction in the number of sample sites. Alternatively, while rapid sampling of flow velocities may improve temporal resolution, too few samples at a given site may result in erroneous information about true flow velocity. A compromise is arrived at so that, by sacrificing completeness of velocity information at each point, only mean velocity is determined, but at many points. As the ultrasound line sweeps through the sector arc, mean velocity is determined throughout the field of view. Sampling frequency and time may be increased by minimizing the scan sector width and depth. This action results in an improvement in the temporal and spatial resolution within the sector but also results in a decrease in the field of view.

Another compromise occurs when the ultrasound lines diverge into the far field of the image and become more separate. At some point in space, they are so far apart that the resultant image would appear broken. To overcome this problem, data from a gate on one line are averaged with data on the adjacent line (Fig. 6-5). This process is repeated for each frame of color data throughout the field of view. The resultant line averaging smooths the appearance of colors in the final display. While this technique provides a more homogeneous image, it should be recognized that data from the far field are less representative of actual flows at that point than data in the near field. This type of processing is also applied to the two-dimensional anatomic data. Decreasing scan depth results in less line averaging and a more accurate representation of flow signals.

Like conventional pulsed-wave Doppler, aliasing may occur in color-flow imaging as well and is dependent on both scan depth and

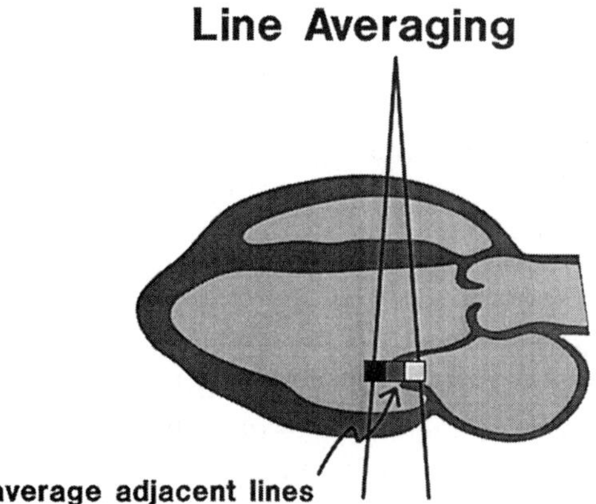

FIGURE 6-5. At the far ranges, gates are separated due to divergence of the radial scan lines. Data from adjacent gates are averaged to smooth the image. Similar methods are used in conventional anatomic scanning for image smoothing and elimination of the scan lines.

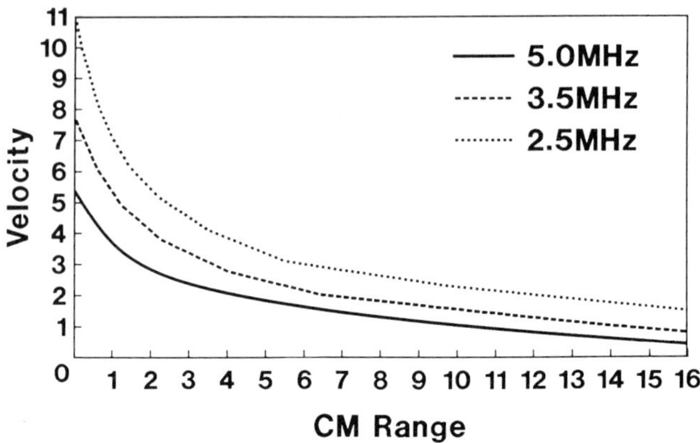

FIGURE 6-6. The maximum velocity able to be recorded without aliasing at any range is a function of the frequency transmitted. *(After materials from Hewlett-Packard, Inc.)*

transducer frequency (Fig. 6-6). Less aliasing is encountered by using lower frequency transducers than higher frequency ones and by scanning at smaller depths than at larger depths. The implications of this fact are significant in clinical scanning. The highest resolution ultrasound scanning is performed with higher frequency transducer systems. Yet, these frequencies have the greatest problem with aliasing. The color correlates of aliasing are indicated by display of progressively brighter and brighter colors as mean velocities rise, until the aliasing point is reached at which there is a reversal of color into the opposite directional channel. At the aliasing point, the brightest hues of red and blue are adjacent. This fact aids the eye in the recognition of aliasing in the final display. While aliasing is a tremendous problem for conventional pulsed-wave Doppler, it is less so for color-flow imaging. Because the aliasing is displayed in two-dimensions as a mosaic, it frequently allows one to readily recognize areas of turbulence associated with disease states. Aliasing is, therefore, frequently used to advantage in the color-flow map since it may dramatically highlight the presence of abnormal high velocities.

The Color-Flow Examination

Intraoperative imaging generally is performed with high-frequency (5.0 MHz) transducers. The technical considerations already cited should be kept in mind when selecting scan depths, sector sizes, and transducer position and angulation. The color-flow examination is accomplished most easily by switching the color control on and off as the operator proceeds with the two-dimensional examination through the various views. Optimal adjustment of the gain setting is essential, as too much gain results in excessive noise in the image and detracts from image quality and interpretability. In most systems, excess gain is readily recognized by the appearance of background noise and distortion in the continuity of flow. Too low a gain setting diminishes sensitivity of the system for detecting small flow disturbances. It also makes large flow distrubances appear artifactually smaller, as the spatial representation of the limits of an abnormal flow jet are entirely dependent on gain. It is quite difficult to make small jets abnormally large by the use of excess gain; however, it is easy to make large jets appear small by the lack of proper gain settings.

Relation to Angiography

One way to conceptualize Doppler color-flow imaging is to recognize its similarity to angiography. It provides a noninvasive angiogram of blood flow, in which the contrast medium is the moving red blood cells, and the detector of this contrast is ultrasound. The complex Doppler ultrasound processing circuitry allows for the detection of movement of these red cells in various directions, forward and backward, through the heart. Doppler color-flow information, however, is obtained and displayed in a cross-sectional image, making the spatial details of flow and anatomy readily recognizable. In effect, Doppler color-flow imaging looks inside the cineangiographic silhouette. However, unlike angiography, Doppler color flow does not depend on dye dilution accumulated over several heart beats. Rather, it displays an abnormal flow jet for each cardiac cycle. Thus, it can display the differing sizes of regurgitant jets dependent on severity. The larger the volume of the regurgitant jet, the larger the size represented on the display. Despite intrinsic differences, qualitative and quantitative estimation of flows by the two techniques yield similar results.[2–7]

Relation to Other Doppler Methods

As color-flow imaging is based on pulsed-wave Doppler principles, it cannot accurately record high velocity information. Because there is no spectral display, precise timing of events is not possible. Also, the time required to process and create the color image further impairs temporal resolution. In addition, aliasing occurs at least as frequently as with conventional pulsed-wave Doppler, and peak velocities used to assess pressure gradients cannot be assessed. Color-flow methods are roughly quantitative concerning the size and direction of abnormal jets. More precise quantitative work, such as derivations of pressure gradients from peak velocity information, remains within the province of continuous-wave Doppler.

Despite these disadvantages, Doppler color-flow imaging, particularly in the intraoperative setting, has advantages over other Doppler modalities. In contrast to conventional pulsed-wave Doppler, normal and abnormal flows are displayed directly on the echocardiographic image and not in a spectral display. When compared with the conventional pulsed-wave Doppler approach, color-flow imaging avoids the tedious mapping techniques necessary with the earlier technique. Thus, for those familiar with two-dimensional imaging, the examination time required for a color-flow study is relatively short compared to the other methods. Simply switching color on and off as the two-dimensional examination is performed can reveal useful information in a short period of time. Despite the machine's increased cost, its ease of use and relatively rapid technical mastery results in considerable savings of time and patient cost.

NORMAL FLOWS

The normal color-flow examination produces many changing colors as the blood flows from chamber to chamber through the cardiac valves. Most normal velocities are relatively low (up to 1.5 m/s) and, even with the high transducer frequencies used in intraoperative imaging, at relatively small scan depths, usually do not result in aliasing. Normal flows are characterized by deep hues, indicating laminar patterns of flow. Changes in direction of flow are signified by a change from red to blue or vice versa. Not only is the color examination useful in characterizing flows, but it also is useful in identifying structures. By switching color on, an echolucent two-dimensional structure can be identified as either containing flow or not, and can be further characterized according to the direction and nature of flow. For example, the entry points of systemic and pulmonary veins into their respective atria can be identified by detection of the color-flow signal.

ABNORMAL FLOWS AND INTRAOPERATIVE UTILITY

Valvular Regurgitation, Mitral

Perhaps the most useful application of intraoperative color-flow imaging is the detection of valvular regurgitation. Mitral regurgitation is recognized as a mosaic-colored turbulent jet of flow in the left atrium, which in real-time is seen to proceed from the left ventricle into the left atrium in systole. The severity of regurgitation can be roughly quantitated based on the width and depth of the regurgitant jet relative to the left atrium (Fig. 6-7). The quantitation correlates well with angiographic estimates of severity.[4,7] Regurgitant jets may flow in any direction and may have virtually any appearance. Color-flow imaging permits localization of the regurgitant jet and can identify whether regurgitation is valvular or perivalvular.

The transesophageal approach is particularly well suited to identification of mitral regurgitation; as the transducer is close to the mitral valve, the direction of ultrasound is nearly parallel to regurgitant flow, and problems of flow masking related to mitral prostheses or calcifica-

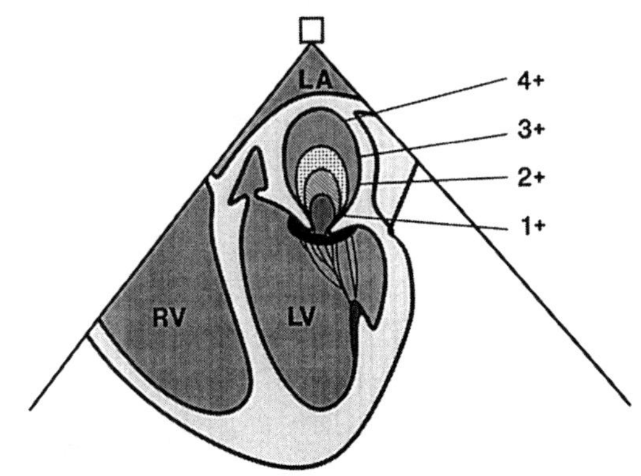

FIGURE 6-7. Estimation of the severity of mitral regurgitation by Doppler color-flow mapping. Both the color jet width and depth are used to render a qualitative estimate of severity. The same principle may be applied in estimating severity of any other regurgitant valve by Doppler color-flow mapping.

tion are not a consideration. An estimation of the severity of mitral regurgitation prior to cardiopulmonary bypass (CPB) helps to determine the type of operation required. In patients with mitral stenosis, a large amount of regurgitation should prompt a mitral valve replacement instead of an open commissurotomy.[8] In patients with ischemic heart disease, a mitral valve repair procedure may either be incorporated into the operative plan if significant mitral regurgitation is detected, or it may be excluded from the operative plan if mitral regurgitation identified preoperatively is not present at the time of the pre-CPB examination.[9] Care needs to be taken to optimize loading conditions and to perform scanning in multiple planes and at optimal gain settings; these factors may affect the assessment of mitral regurgitation. For small and eccentrically directed jets, extra time is required to be sure of proper identification and characterization.

Post-CPB mitral regurgitation can also be assessed. Following mitral valve replacement or repair, echocardiographic assessment of residual regurgitation is useful to assess the adequacy of the operation. The method is superior to other techniques of assessing mitral competency, such as left atrial pressure waveforms, direct palpation, or saline injection into the left ventricle.[3,4,8] Significant residual regurgitation identifies patients at higher risk for postoperative morbidity or mortality.[8]

Direct epicardial scanning is also useful in assessing mitral regurgitation both before and after CPB. While it permits scanning in a greater variety of planes, however, its intrusion into the operative field and its potential for masking the regurgitant flow signal because of echogenic mitral prostheses or mitral calcification potentially limit the use of this technique compared to transesophageal scanning.

Valvular Regurgitation, Aortic

Almost all of the previous comments also apply to the detection and quantification of aortic insufficiency. Aortic regurgitant jets may be small and narrow and are characterized as mosaic-colored flow seen to proceed from the aorta into the left ventricle in diastole. As the aortic valve lies more anterior to the mitral valve and typically in a plane at right angles to the mitral valve, imaging from the transesophageal approach may be more difficult. Presence of a mitral prosthesis may result in masking of the flow signal of aortic regurgitation when assessed transesophageally. When these considerations apply, direct epicardial scanning may be superior to transesophageal scanning. As is the case for mitral regurgitation, the aortic regurgitant jet may be precisely localized as valvular or perivalvular. Transesophageal examination is particularly well suited to the assessment of aortic dissection, as it is possible to visualize flow within the true and false lumens, as well as any accompanying aortic insufficiency.

Valvular Regurgitation, Right Sided

As with the left valves, tricuspid and pulmonic regurgitant jets may be found in any size, spatial configuration, and direction. Because the right valves are in an anterior location, transesophageal imaging is not well suited to assessment of regurgitant flow. In this case, direct epicardial imaging is superior. Typically, tricuspid regurgitation is recognized as a mosaic-colored jet in systole, proceeding from the right ventricle into the right atrium. Pulmonic insufficiency typically is manifest in the epicardial basal short-axis view, in which the flamelike regurgitant jet is seen in diastole to proceed from the pulmonary artery into the right ventricle.

Valvular Stenosis

Doppler color-flow imaging methods can identify the presence of certain valvular stenotic jets. Stenotic flows are characterized by mosaic-colored, turbulent jets directed in an anterograde direction. No specific characteristics in the color display of stenotic flows, however, help quantitate the severity of valvular obstruction. With some systems, color-flow imaging permits spatial location of the direction of a jet. Image-directed continuous-wave Doppler interrogation can then be positioned at an optimum angle to flow for precise measurement of peak velocity data.

Doppler color-flow examination immediately before the operation, either from the epicardial or transesophageal approach, usually furnishes no additional information to the routine preoperative evaluation of patients who are undergoing operations to treat valvular stenosis.[8,10] However, post-CPB examination may be useful in a variety of circumstances. As previously indicated, a proper assessment of valvular stenosis is best accomplished in the intraoperative setting with image-directed continuous-wave Doppler capabilities. In this manner, peak and mean transvalvular gradients across valvular prostheses and across sites of valve repair, valvotomy, and commissurotomy may be determined as an assessment of the efficacy of the operation. Left ventricular outflow obstruction occurs in as many as 10% of patients after mitral valve repair,[11] and, if recognized intraoperatively, should prompt revision of the repair or placement of a mitral valve prosthesis (Color plate 1).[8] This situation may be identified by Doppler color-flow imaging as subaortic, anterograde turbulence associated with systolic anterior motion of the mitral valve apparatus. Indirect information about the efficacy of relief of valvular stenosis may be provided by assessment of other intracardiac flows. For example, after right ventricular outflow patching to ameliorate tetralogy of Fallot, if the direction of the flow across the ventricular septal defect continues to be from right to left, then elevated right ventricular pressures persist, and inadequate relief of pulmonic stenosis is indicated.[12]

Valvular Prostheses

Imaging of flow through prosthetic valves is possible and may be of great help in assessing the proper working status of these valves. As previously indicated, Doppler color-flow imaging performed intraoperatively may be particularly useful in the immediate post-CPB assessment of both prosthetic valve regurgitation and stenosis.[8] Furthermore, color-flow imaging provides a means for easy spatial identification of flows that occur either through prosthetic valves or for those that are periprosthetic. Assessment of prosthetic valve stenosis is more difficult but may be aided by image-directed continuous-wave Doppler.

Congenital Disorders

Intraoperative Doppler color-flow imaging is extremely useful when used during operations for congenital heart disease.[12–15] Epicardial imaging appears to be better suited for routine application in most instances. Available sizes of transesophageal probes make their placement in small children difficult and more hazardous. Furthermore, the complexity of many congenital conditions requires imaging in a greater variety of planes than those generally afforded by transesophageal imaging.

Artrial septal defects may be encountered in both adults and children. Both transesophageal and epicardial imaging reveal a mosaic-appearing jet of flow traversing the interatrial septum. The direction of flow is dictated by the relative right and left atrial pressures. Ventricular septal defects may similarly be detected as flow jets traversing the interventricular septum (Color plate 2). Doppler color-flow imaging permits spatial localization of these defects, an ability which not only facilitates the point of initial repair but also may guide the location of further repair if post-CPB residual shunting is detected. As is true for post-CPB defects identified by transesophageal Doppler color-flow imaging in adults, post-CPB residual defects identified by epicardial imaging in children who are undergoing operations for congenital heart disease identify a group of patients at higher risk for postoperative morbidity and mortality.[13]

Miscellaneous Applications

Intraoperative Doppler color-flow imaging may help identify and localize flows within the coronary arteries and bypass grafts.[16] Such an assessment may permit an evaluation of the adequacy of flow through these arteries and may localize native arteries to which bypass grafts are to be placed. Doppler color-flow imaging is a well-recognized modality for the identification of aortic dissections.[17] In the intraoperative setting, the technique provides a means for the assessment of the adequacy of repair after surgery and gives a pre-CPB assessment of the extent of the dissection.

CONCLUSION

While intraoperative echocardiography has long been recognized as a useful tool in patients who are undergoing cardiac surgery,[18] the recent introduction of Doppler color-flow imaging has been instrumental in its widespread application. The technique, whether applied epicardially or transesophageally, is safe and rapid and provides reliable and useful diagnostic information. The simultaneous assessment of real-time cardiac structure and flow provided by Doppler color-flow imaging is an invaluable aid in the pre-CPB formulation of surgical plan and post-CPB assessment of surgical results.

References

1. Kisslo J, Adams DB, Belkin RN: Doppler Color Flow Imaging. New York, Churchill Livingstone, 1988
2. Miyatake K, Izumi S, Okamoto M et al: Semiquantitative grading of severity of mitral regurgitation by real-time two-dimensional Doppler flow imaging technique. J Am Coll Cardiol 7:82, 1986
3. Czer LSC, Maurer G, Bolger AF et al: Intraoperative evaluation of mitral regurgitation by Doppler color flow mapping. Circulation 76 (suppl):108, 1987

4. Maurer G, Czer LSC, Chaux A et al: Intraoperative Doppler color flow mapping for assessment of valve repair for mitral regurgitation. Am J Cardiol 60:333, 1987
5. Helmcke R, Nanda NC, Hsiung MC et al: Color Doppler assessment of mitral regurgitation with orthogonal planes. Circulation 75:175, 1987
6. Spain MG, Smith MD, Grayburn PA et al: Quantitative assessment of mitral regurgitation by Doppler color flow imaging: Angiographic and hemodynamic correlations. J Am Coll Cardiol 13:585, 1989
7. Omoto R, Yokote Y, Takamota S et al: The development of real-time two-dimensional Doppler echocardiography and its clinical significance in acquired valvular diseases with special reference to the evaluation of valvular regurgitation. Jpn Heart J :325, 1984
8. Sheikh K, de Bruijn N, Rankin JS et al: The utility of transesophageal echocardiography and Doppler color flow imaging in patients undergoing cardiac valve operations. J Am Coll Cardiol 15:363, 1990
9. Sheikh K, Bengtson J, Rankin J, de Bruijn N, Kisslo J: Pre-bypass transesophageal color flow mapping used to guide surgery for ischemic mitral regurgitation. Circulation 80:II-424, 1989
10. Sheikh K, de Bruijn N, Rankin J, Clements F, Kisslo J: Utility of intraoperative transesophageal echocardiography in valve and coronary bypass operations. Circulation 80:II-338, 1989
11. Galler M, Kronzon I, Slater J et al: Long-term follow-up after mitral valve reconstruction: Incidence of postoperative left ventricular outflow obstruction. Circulation 75 (suppl):99, 1986
12. Ungerleider R, Greeley W, Sheikh K et al: Routine use of intraoperative epicardial echo and Doppler color flow imaging to guide and evaluate repair of congenital heart lesions: A prospective study. J Thorac Cardiovasc Surg 100:297, 1990
13. Ungerleider RM, Greeley WJ, Sheikh KH, Kern FH, Kisslo JA, Sabiston DC: The use of intraoperative echo with Doppler color flow imaging to predict outcome after repair of congenital cardiac defects. Ann Surg 210:526, 1989
14. Ungerleider RM, Kisslo JA, Greeley WJ, Van Trigt P, Sabiston DC: Intraoperative pre-bypass and post-bypass epicardial color flow imaging in the repair of atrioventricular septal defects. J Thorac Cardiovasc Surg 98:90, 1989
15. Takamoto S, Kyo S, Adachi H, Matsumura M, Yokote Y, Omoto R: Intraoperative color flow mapping by real-time two-dimensional Doppler echocardiography for evaluation of valvular and congenital heart disease and vascular disease. J Thorac Cardiovasc Surg 90:802, 1985
16. Pearce FB, Sheikh KH, de Bruijn NP, Kisslo J: Imaging of the coronary arteries by transesophageal echocardiography. J Am Society of Echocardiography 2:276, 1989
17. Erbel R, Borner N, Steller D, Brunier J, Thelen M, Pfeiffer C: Detection of aortic dissection by transesophageal echocardiography. Br Heart J 58:45, 1987
18. Johnson ML, Holmes JH, Spangler RD, Paton BR: Usefulness of echocardiography in patients undergiong mitral valve surgery. J Thorac Cardiovasc Surg 64:922, 1972

Norbert P. de Bruijn
Fiona M. Clements

7 Evaluation of Valvular Dysfunction and Repair by Echocardiography

Since the development of Doppler echocardiographic technology, ultrasound has played an increasingly important role in the evaluation of the anatomy and function of the heart valves. The two classic modalities of Doppler echocardiography are continuous-wave Doppler, which allows the user to measure blood flow velocity within the heart and blood vessels without being limited by a maximum measurable velocity, but it restricts the physician by its inability to precisely locate the position at which this velocity is being measured; and pulsed-wave Doppler, which does enable the observer to precisely locate the spot at which the blood-flow velocity is being measured, but it has a limited maximum blood-flow velocity that can be measured due to the inherent limitations of the technique.

In spite of these limitations, both techniques are extremely useful in defining pathophysiologic conditions of the heart valves. Echocardiography has been revolutionized, however, by the recent development of a new Doppler modality: Doppler color-flow imaging, a pulsed-wave Doppler technique that translates the difficult-to-interpret information from the classically measured waveforms that represent blood-flow velocity, into a color map that represents blood-flow velocities throughout the heart. This technique is similar to a cineangiogram, in which the contrast medium is the moving red blood cells and the detector of this contrast is ultrasound. This electronically complicated but generally operator-friendly technology allows the user to assess at a glance the direction and velocity of the blood flow as well as the presence of abnormal jets. The development of this technology made Doppler imaging a practical option in the operating room. This chapter briefly outlines the basics of Doppler color-flow mapping and discusses its actual uses in the operating room to evaluate valve function.

HOW IS A COLOR IMAGE CREATED?

For an explanation of Doppler technology and physics, see Chapters 2 and 10.

Doppler color-flow imaging is based on pulsed-wave Doppler principles but is a refinement and enhancement of this technique. This section explores how pulsed-wave Doppler is used to create a color flow image and examines some of the limitations of the technique.[1]

One of the most important limiting factors in the process of making a color-flow image is time. A two-dimensional ultrasound imaging system is already working hard: ultrasound pulses are transmitted, reflected from the cardiac structures, and received back. This process is repeated line by line through the entire sector arc that comprises hundreds of lines. To have the image appear as though it is continuously moving, the entire image must be updated thirty times per second. This fact means that large amounts of data must be processed in a short time.

If the system is kept this busy to create a two-dimensional image alone, how can it also rapidly take Doppler samples all over the image field and translate them into a color map? Doppler color-flow imaging is based on what is known as *multigate* Doppler: a burst of ultrasound is sent into the tissue, and, subsequently, the echo transducer rapidly receives the reflected ultrasound at x incremental times, x being the number of "gates" along a given line of interrogation. Thus, the Doppler system receives data from the nearest gate first and from the gate farthest away last. The number of gates along a line can be in the hundreds (250–500). In color-flow imaging, the transducer scans the whole sector arc, line for line, with this multigated technique and translates the blood-flow velocity data into a color, which is assigned to the appropriate gate and displayed. This whole process takes place in a 30th of a second. The process becomes more complex considering that, even in the case of normal (laminar), flow, many different velocities may be measurable within a single gate at a particular time, and the system has to calculate, or rather estimate, a mean velocity.

This estimate of mean velocity in each gate represents another compromise in comparison to pulsed-wave Doppler. In the latter technique, Fast Fourier Transform is used to analyze the velocity data. This method is too time consuming for Doppler color-flow imaging; the analysis here is performed by a much cruder technique called *autocorrelation* or *instantaneous frequency estimation.* The details of these analysis techniques go far beyond the scope of this chapter.

In addition to measuring the frequency shift and calculating a mean velocity, the system must eliminate some of the noise that is part of the received echos. This process is known as *clutter rejection* or *combing.*

DOPPLER TECHNICALITIES

The most important of the technicalities of Doppler imaging is the phenomenon of *frequency aliasing,* usually called just *aliasing.* Aliasing occurs when the blood-flow velocity to be measured exceeds the rate at which the pulsed-wave Doppler system can record it properly. In classic pulsed-wave Doppler, the result is that the top of the velocity curve is cut off and displayed in the opposite channel (see Chapter 10). In Doppler color-flow imaging, aliasing results in color reversal. The color red (representing flow towards the transducer) becomes blue, and blue (representing flow away from the transducer) becomes red. As the blood-flow velocity increses, the red (or blue) becomes brighter and brighter until the Nyquist limit is reached (see Chapter 2), at which point the color reverses into the brightest shade of blue (respectively red). Actually, in Doppler color-flow imaging, aliasing may help the observer recognize (abnormally) high blood-flow velocities because the color reversal stands out quite remarkably. Unlike normal pulsed-wave Doppler, aliasing in color Doppler does not necessarily indicate abnormally high blood-flow velocity; the pulse-repetition frequency is so relatively low due to the large amount of data that has to be processed within a short time.

Even more than in pulsed-wave Doppler, it is important, therefore, in color Doppler to work in the near field and with the lowest possible transducer frequency. The choice in transesophageal ultrasound transducers is limited, however.

Another feature of most Doppler color systems is their ability to detect and display blood-flow velocity variance. In laminar (normal) blood flow, the spectrum of measurable velocities is narrow and the mean blood flow velocity is close to the peak velocity. In turbulent flow, however, blood flows at many different velocities, so the velocity spectrum is wide. The variance algorithms detect the spectral broadening present in these abnormal flows and express the amount of variance by adding green to the blue and red display.

TRANSESOPHAGEAL ECHOCARDIOGRAPHY AND THE VALVES

With knowledge of two-dimensional echocardiography and Doppler color-flow imaging, the valves in the heart suitable for evaluation by these techniques can be examined. In most patients, all cardiac valves, mitral, aortic, tricuspid, and pulmonic, can be visualized. Nevertheless, not all of these valves are suitable for evaluation with transesophageal echocardiography (TEE). The mitral valve is close to the esophageal ultrasound transducer, and, invariably, this position provides superb image quality. The blood flow through this valve is virtually parallel to the ultrasound beam, and, thus, high-quality Doppler imaging is possible as well. The mitral valve is without a doubt the most suitable for transesophageal imaging. In most instances, the aortic valve can be imaged only in a short-axis plane (with the standard single-plane esophageal transducers), and almost invariably the image quality is high. The direction of the blood flow in this plane, however, is perpendicular to the ultrasound beam so that the Doppler information is of limited use. The left ventricular outflow tract can be imaged well in all patients, and the angle of the blood flow with the ultrasound beam is rather small, so that aortic regurgitant jets can most often be imaged well. The right valves pose a problem: the tricuspid and pulmonic valves are anterior structures and, thus, rather far from the transducer. Both two-dimensional imaging and color-flow imaging are often suboptimal; these valves are better approached with epicardial echocardiography.

The Mitral Valve

Under normal conditions, mitral valve competence is maintained by a complex interaction of the five components of its morphology and function: (1) the ventricular wall, (2) the fibrous annulus, (3) the papillary muscles, (4) the chordae tendineae, and (5) the valve leaflets. Derangement of any of these components may cause valve dysfunction.[2]

Embryologically, the mitral valve is initially quadricuspid. As development continues, the accessory or commissural scallops or cusps fuse with and become part of the lateral aspects of the posterior leaflet.

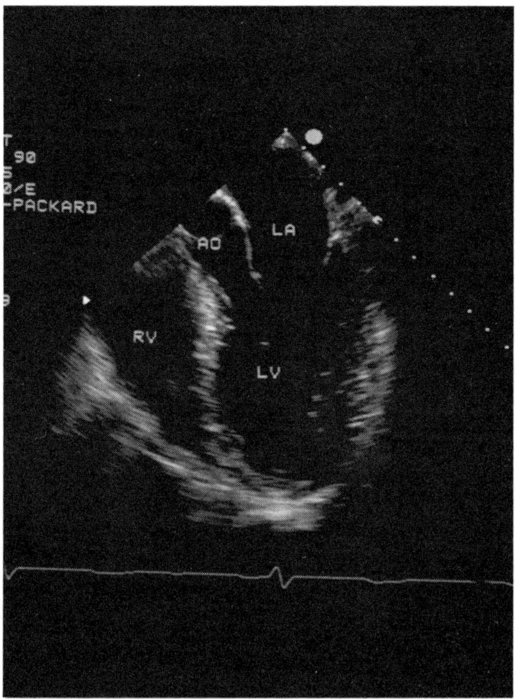

FIGURE 7-1. Transesophageal long-axis view of the heart in diastole. The mitral valve is open, and the relative length of the anterior and posterior leaflets can easily be appreciated. *AO*, aorta; *LA*, left atrium; *RV*, right ventricle; *LV*, left ventricle.

Persistence of these fetal commissural cusps, especially at the posterior commissure, may produce scalloping of the lateral aspect of the posterior leaflet or minor posterior leaflet defects. In most adults, however, only two leaflets are evident: a broad anterior leaflet and a narrow posterior leaflet. In spite of the fact that the anterior leaflet is broader, the surface area of each leaflet is almost identical because of the annular attachment of the posterior leaflet, which is almost twice as long as that of the anterior leaflet (Fig. 7-1).

The papillary muscles arise from the ventricular walls, approximately two thirds of the distance toward the apex. The anterolateral papillary muscle is single in the majority of patients, whereas the posteromedial one has multiple heads. The anterolateral muscle is supplied by branches of the proximal anterior descending or circumflex coronary artery and has a more abundant blood supply than the posteromedial muscle, which is supplied by a single coronary artery, usually one of the posterolateral branches of the right coronary artery.

Three orders of chordae tendineae are recognized: first order chordae originate at the apices of the papillary muscles and insert into the free edges of the leaflets; second order chordae also originate at the apices of the papillary muscles, but they insert on the ventricular side of the leaflets, about 1 to 3 mm from the free edge; tertiary chordae originate from the ventricular walls and insert near the basal aspect of mainly the posterior leaflet. The point that the valve coapts is not the free edge but is located a short distance proximally on the leaflet so that the leaflets coapt along a considerable area of their atrial surface. Because the point where they coapt is below the mitral annulus, the

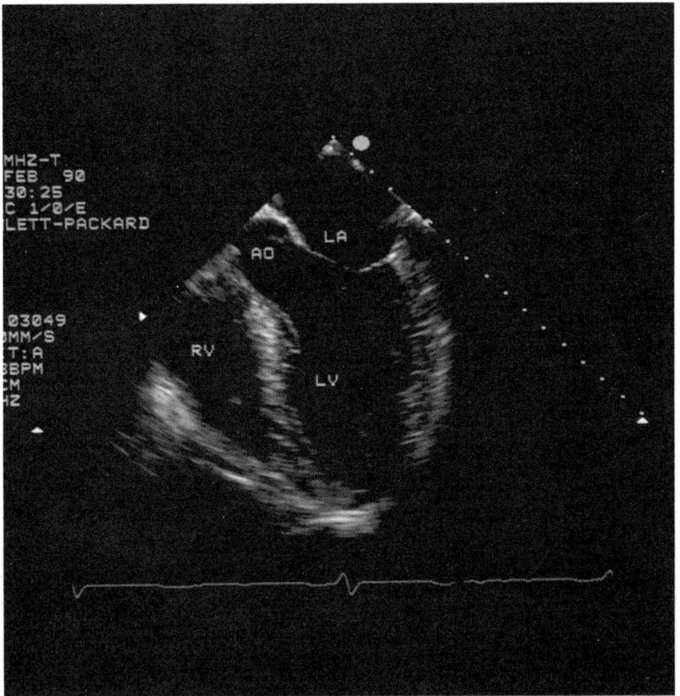

FIGURE 7-2. Transesophageal long-axis view of the heart in systole. Note that the apposition point of the mitral is located in the left ventricle. *AO,* aorta; *LA,* left atrium; *RV,* right ventricle; *LV,* left ventricle.

closed valve has a chevron shape on a long-axis, two-dimensional cross section.

In a long-axis plane, it is obvious that the anterior leaflet is considerably longer from its annular origin to the tip than the posterior leaflet (Fig. 7-2). The anterior leaflet can be seen to be continuous with the posterior wall of the aortic root. The continuation of the left atrial wall at the atrioventricular sulcus can be seen to appear to give rise to the posterior mitral leaflet. It can also be seen that the anterior leaflet is more mobile than its posterior counterpart.

In most patients, the subvalvular apparatus can be visualized as well, provided one uses appropriate (low) gain settings. Both the origin and insertion points of some of the chordae can frequently be appreciated.

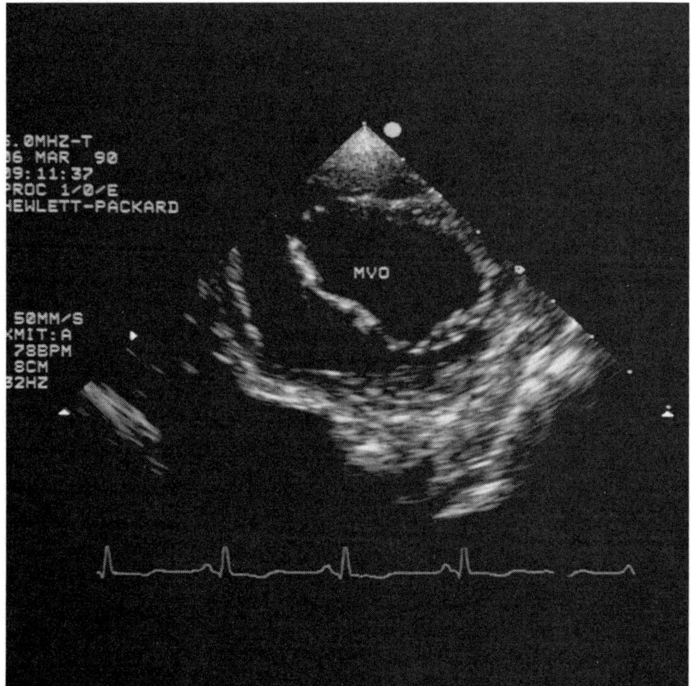

FIGURE 7-3. Transesophageal short-axis view of the left ventricle with the mitral valve in the open position *(MVO)*. The leaflet closest to the apex of the sector is the posterior leaflet. Its long attachment in relation to the anterior leaflet can be seen easily.

In a short-axis view, the mitral valve appears as a fish mouth (Fig. 7-3).The leaflet closest to the apex of the sector is the posterior leaflet, and sometimes scalloping can be seen in this leaflet. Although Doppler studies are performed best in a long-axis plane to line up the ultrasound beam with the direction of the blood flow, additional information about the location of abnormal jets may be obtained in this short-axis plane with Doppler color-flow imaging.

Mitral valve pathology often can be partially recognized by two-dimensional imaging alone (Fig. 7-4). Myxomatous degeneration of the mitral valve is most commonly associated with leaflet prolapse, chordal rupture, or both and is often accompanied by annular dilatation. On the other hand, rheumatic involvement produces leaflet retraction, fibrotic thickening, and calcification that show up as enhanced echo

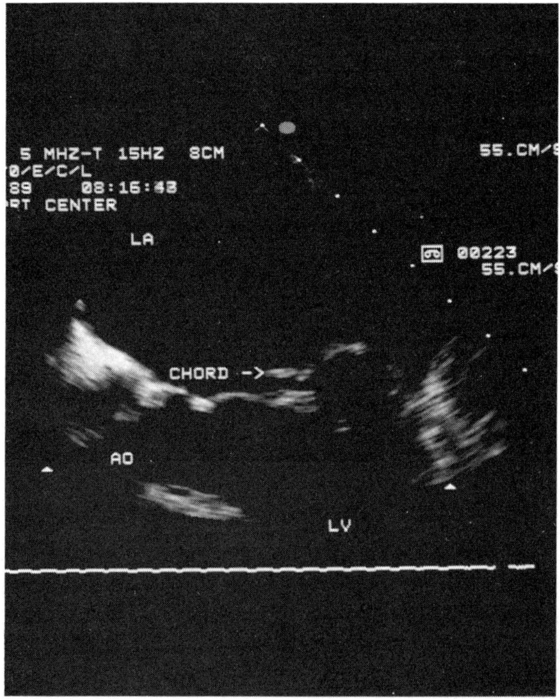

FIGURE 7-4. Transesophageal close-up view of the mitral valve in systole. The posterior leaflet can be seen to prolapse into the left atrium *(LA)*, and a broken chord *(arrow)* is readily apparent.

density. In ischemic mitral regurgitation, the valve may show prolapse but frequently actually has a remarkably normal appearance.

Doppler color-flow imaging allows us to assess the presence and, to a certain extent, the severity of mitral regurgitation or mitral stenosis (Color plate 3). The most useful plane to detect either stenosis or regurgitation is the long-axis two- or four-chamber view. Almost always aliasing is seen, owing to the increased blood-flow velocity in the jet. Most of the time turbulence is also present. The process of estimating the amount of mitral regurgitation is somewhat controversial, and a number of systems have been proposed in an attempt to quantitate regurgitation. "Eyeballing" the size and configuration of the jet is as good a system as any, provided the observer has a fair amount of experience. An experienced observer can consistently classify mitral regurgitation in three or four classes of severity. Trivial amounts of mitral regurgitation are often seen by TEE in normal patients.

Regurgitant and stenotic jets should not be evaluated in a vacuum; many factors influence the size, direction, and velocity of abnormal jets. Important considerations are the pressure gradient between the left atrium and the left ventricle, the size and compliance of the left atrium, the size and configuration of the mitral orifice, the volume of the regurgitating blood, preload and afterload, the presence or absence of sinus rhythm, and the heart rate.

During the examination of a valve, it is important to remember that we are examining thin, two-dimensional planes and the ultrasound beam must be made to scan the entire depth of the valve to not overlook localized pathology.

Imaging mitral stenosis is more problematic than imaging regurgitation because the stenotic jet is by definition located in the far field. Also, the mitral valve is frequently heavily calcified, a fact which results in a degree of "masking" of the image distal to the valve and produces reverberations that degrade the quality of the image.

Utility of Echo/Doppler Examination of the Mitral Valve

Transesophageal Doppler color-flow imaging, in contrast to plain two-dimensional imaging, requires expensive equipment, the expensive additional training of anesthesiologists, and the back-up services of a cardiologist with a background in transesophageal and intraoperative ultrasound techniques. All of these requirements result in an increase in cost to the patient and the health care system in an era in which we are desperately trying to reduce cost. Is this expense justified?

In an effort to answer this question, we assessed the utility of intraoperative TEE in 154 patients out of 686 who were undergoing cardiac valve surgery.[3] All patients had two-dimensional transesophageal ultrasound exams before and after cardiopulmonary bypass and surgical repair or replacement of the affected valve. One hundred and three patients also had Doppler color-flow imaging performed at these times.

Surgical decisions based on the use of TEE in the operating room were categorized as: 1) unsuspected findings before initiation of cardiopulmonary bypass that either assisted or changed the planned operation, 29 of the 154 patients (19%); 2) identification of inadequate initial operative results leading to further surgery, 10 of the 154 patients (6%); 3) pharmacologic support instituted because of postbypass ventricular dysfunction, 13 of the 154 patients (8%). The greatest impact of TEE was observed with the use concomitant two-dimensional and Doppler color-flow imaging in patients who were undergoing mitral valve surgery. Postbypass TEE assessment of surgical results and ventricular function was related to postoperative prognosis. Of 95 patients judged to have adequate valvular function after surgical replacement or repair, 14 (15%) experienced major postoperative complications, and 5 (5%) died. In comparison, of 7 patients judged to have residual valvular defects of moderate degree, 6 (86%) had postoperative complications,

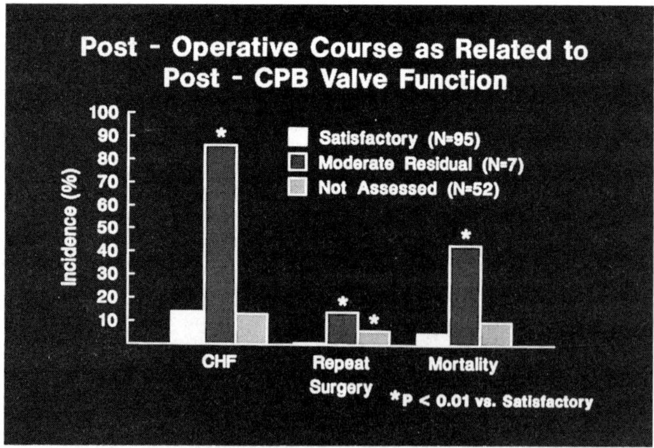

FIGURE 7-5. The effects of the adequacy of valve repair on some outcome variables.

and 4 (43%) died (Fig. 7-5). Both of these differences were statistically significant. Similarly, of 131 patients with preserved left ventricular function by TEE, 12 (9%) had major complications, and 7 (5%) died (Fig. 7-6). In contrast, of 23 patients with reduced ventricular function immediately after cardiopulmonary bypass, 17 (73%) experienced major complications, and 6 (26%) died. These differences were also statistically and clinically significant. This study indicates that intraoperative TEE, especially when Doppler color-flow imaging is being used, is useful to formulate the surgical plan, to assess the result before the patient leaves the operating room so that immediate corrective action can be taken, and to identify patients at risk for significant postoperative complications. If these initial results are borne out by other studies,[4] this tool will prove cost effective and will help to prevent serious perioperative misery.

The Aortic Valve

The aortic valve can be well imaged in a cross-sectional or short-axis view but less successfully in a long-axis plane, at least with most of the available single-plane esophageal transducers. Before using Doppler color-flow mapping to evaluate the functional status of the valve, the plain, two-dimensional image should be examined to look at the three valve cusps that form the familiar Mercedes-Benz sign. These cusps

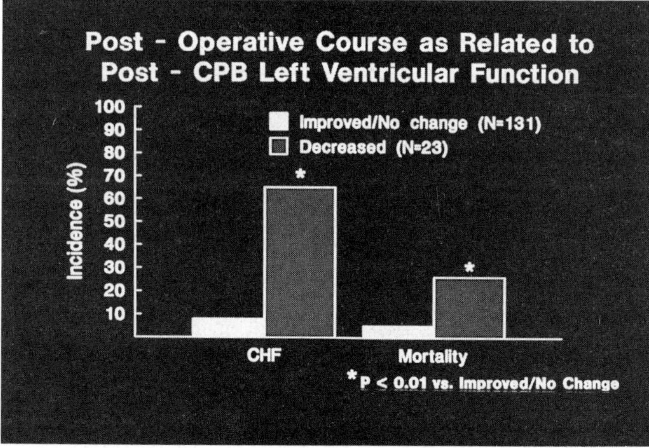

FIGURE 7-6. The effects of left ventricular function after valve procedures on some outcome variables.

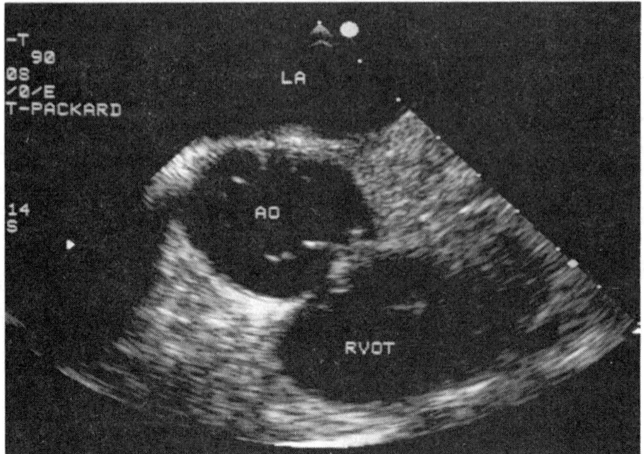

FIGURE 7-7A. A short-axis transesophageal view of the aortic valve during systole; the cusps can be seen to open well to the periphery.

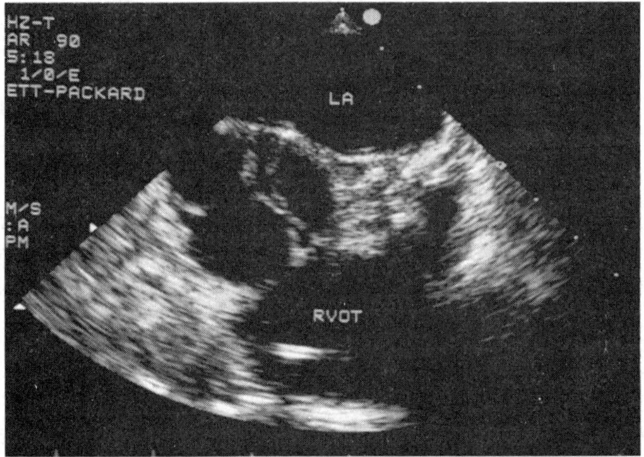

FIGURE 7-7B. The aortic valve during diastole shows the typical Mercedes-Benz configuration.

should be thin and should coapt during diastole while opening well to the periphery of the aorta during systole (Fig. 7-7 A, B). Occasionally the right or left coronary cusp can be seen to prolapse into the left ventricular outflow tract. With the single plane available on most esophageal ultrasound transducers, prolapse of the noncoronary cusp gener-

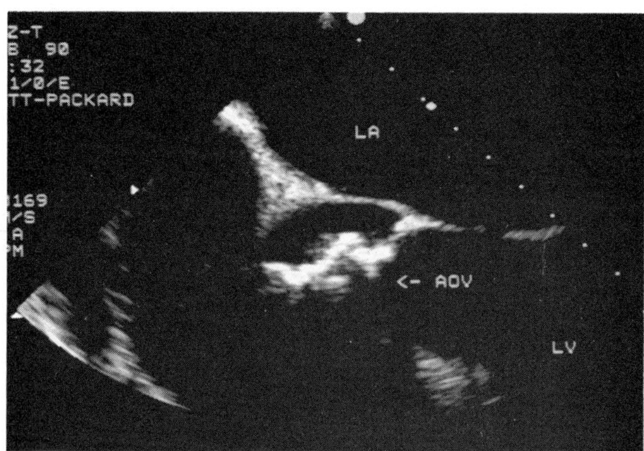

FIGURE 7-8. This aortic valve shows bright echoes *(arrow)*, indicative of calcification, on the valve cusps with a significant amount of "masking" behind the valve because ultrasound does not penetrate calcium well.

ally cannot be evaluated. Deposits of calcium on the valve appear as bright echoes, which are usually irregular and are often associated with valve thickening and poor motion (Fig. 7-8). The sight of this enhanced echo-density on the valve cusps makes it impossible to attribute this increase in density to calcification; fibrosis or other causes may be responsible for this phenomenon.

Vegetations appear as irregular and sometimes quite large growths attached to the valve cusps; they may oscillate to either side of the valve during systole and diastole. They do not generally appear as bright or as fixed as calcific deposits, and they do not cause "shadowing." An abnormal valve provides a clue as to what may be expected in terms of stenotic or regurgitant blood flow. With the transducer behind the left atrium, therefore, a four- or two-chamber image is sought, and then the transducer is made to angle slightly anteriorly to bring the left ventricular outflow tract into view. With the mitral and aortic valves displayed next to each other in this view, systole and diastole are indicated by the alternate opening and closing of the two valves. On the black and white, two-dimensional image, regurgitant flow through the aortic valve may be seen to strike the anterior mitral valve leaflet that is open during diastole by observing a characteristic flutter. The presence of an aortic regurgitant jet can then be confirmed by Doppler color-flow mapping (Color plate 4). Often aortic regurgitant jets can be seen to arise from the central point of the valve where the leaflets are supposed to coapt. At other times, an eccentric jet may be seen passing through a torn or prolapsed cusp. A short-axis image may then help to determine which cusp is torn, which cusp is prolapsing, or where, in the case of a prosthetic valve, a paravalvular leak is located. As with the mitral valve, the general unavailability of biplane images restricts the ability to locate some of these defects as precisely as may be desired.

Because a jet may be narrow and unidirectional, it is also important to look around, as far as possible, to be sure not to miss any regurgitant flow. Such jets may have a high velocity, in excess of $3\ m \cdot s^{-1}$, and cause aliasing with Doppler color-flow mapping, which, as previously noted, actually helps to identify them. A greater problem arises in deciding the significance of a jet. When aortic regurgitation is severe, more of the left ventricle fills in diastole and generally the "base" of the jet is wider than in the case of mild aortic regurgitation.

Several attempts have been made to quantitate aortic insufficiency with Doppler color-flow mapping, comparing it to aortography, which is itself only a semiquantitative measure. The area of the turbulence, the overall length of the jet extending back into the left ventricle, and the width of the jet have all been used to gauge the severity of aortic insufficiency. It seems that the best correlation with angiographic grading is made with a measure of the short-axis area of the jet or the width of the jet at its origin in the left ventricular outflow tract. At its origin, the jet is fairly well defined, so that either its diameter or area can be measured from a freeze frame. Elsewhere, the area of the jet may be affected by the mitral inflow and by ventricular mixing. The area and the length of the jet are also susceptible to variation with different imaging planes and to loading conditions; the size of the jet at its origin probably correlates more closely with the size of the valvular defect. In the case of the aortic valve, as with the mitral valve, "eyeballing" by an experienced observer is probably as good as any of these semiquantitative measures.

Aortic stenosis is a problem. Even with the use of chest wall echocardiography, it is often difficult to delineate the forward jet of aortic stenosis into the aortic root with color-flow methodology. With TEE, it is virtually impossible to image the forward jet, owing to the inability to obtain a long-axis view of the aortic valve and the aortic root. In general, the best procedure is to observe a large amount of turbulence in a short-axis plane just above the valve, suggesting the presence of aortic stenosis. What can be seen frequently is the systolic flow in the left ventricular outflow tract, just before the blood exits through the aortic valve. Flow in the left ventricular outflow tract appears as a narrow jet, as if the red blood cells were "lining up" to pass through the narrowed aortic valve.

Dynamic subvalvular stenosis is seen in idiopathic hypertrophic subaortic stenosis. This condition is accompanied by so-called systolic anterior motion of the anterior leaflet of the mitral valve, which is thought to occur as a consequence of the high velocity flow through the left ventricular outflow tract narrowed by the subaortic stenosis. Venturi forces that result from this high velocity flow are thought to cause a venturi effect, pulling the anterior mitral leaflet toward the interventricular septum. This traction on the mitral leaflet in systole may be bad enough to cause significant mitral regurgitation. The subvalvular obstruction causes high blood-flow velocity and turbulence in the left ventricular outflow tract, conditions which are obvious on the color map.

Intraoperative imaging of the outflow tract in idiopathic hypertrophic subaortic stenosis may help guide the surgeon in the resection of part of the interventricular septum and may be useful in immediate, intraoperative assessment of the efficacy of the myomectomy.

The increasing desire among surgeons recently has been to try to repair aortic valves instead of replacing them. In the case of mitral repairs, it is possible to check the efficacy of the repair in the relaxed, open heart, albeit this possibility is not very reliable. In aortic valve repairs, this possibility does not exist at all, and the only good way to assess the repair appears to be intraoperative echocardiography.

Two types of repairs are performed on a regular basis. In patients with a moderate amount of aortic valve calcification, a procedure known as *CUSA* has been done. This methodology uses ultrasound to "vibrate" the calcium deposits of the valve cusps. Generally, the method has proven to be quite effective to "clean up" the valve cusps; enthusiasm for the procedure is waning a bit, however, because of the relatively large number of patients who come back with aortic regurgitation, probably caused by scarring of the valve cusps. The second procedure was developed by Cosgrove as a repair for aortic regurgitation. This procedure is mainly used for patients in whom annular dilatation has caused the cusps to be pulled apart. It consists of placing sutures through the three valve commissures to pull the cusps together.

Both procedures require the valve to be free of significant residual regurgitation; this condition can be ascertained by using Doppler color-flow imaging of the left ventricular outflow tract. Although not as spectacularly useful as in mitral valve surgery, intraoperative echocardiography caused a modification in the planned surgical procedure in 9% of cases of aortic valve surgery in a recent study. Even in aortic valve replacements, significant residual aortic regurgitation due to inability to properly seat the valve prosthesis or due to malfunctioning of the leaflets is not an extremely rare occurrence. Diagnosing prosthetic valvular regurgitation intraoperatively may prevent the need to return the patient to the operating room for correction of this residual defect at a later date.

References

1. Kisslo JA, Adams DB, Belkin RN: Doppler Color Flow Imaging. New York, Churchill Livingstone, 1988
2. Roberts WC, Perloff JK: Mitral valve disease: A clinicopathologic survey of the conditions causing the mitral valve to function abnormally. Ann Int Med 77:939, 1972
3. Sheikh KH, de Bruijn NP, Rankin JS et al: The utility of transesophageal echocardiography and Doppler color flow imaging in patients undergoing cardiac valve operations. J Am Coll Cardiol 15:363, 1990
4. Rankin JS, St J Hickey M, Smith LR et al: Current management of mitral valve incompetence associated with coronary artery disease. J Cardiovasc Surg (Torino) 4:25, 1989

William J. Greeley
Ross M. Ungerleider

8 Echocardiography During Surgery for Congenital Heart Disease

The broad spectrum of defects and the complexity of operations confound the intraoperative anesthetic and surgical management of patients who are undergoing surgical repair of congenital heart disease. Many elements during the repair influence overall outcome. The most critical element in achieving successful repair is performance of a technically accurate and efficient surgical correction. To obtain these results, a clear description of the anatomy and of how these anatomic variations affect physiology is necessary. This information enables formulation of the most appropriate surgical procedure. Furthermore, after completion of the reconstruction, it is important to be able to evaluate the quality of the repair to insure that these patients leave the operating room with the best result possible. Because intracardiac repair radically alters blood-flow patterns and cardiac structure, the effect of the surgery on cardiac function and physiology is also important to determine.

Intraoperative assessment during and after surgery for congenital heart disease has been restricted to visual inspection of the heart and isolated pressure measurements, usually central venous pressure with occasional use of transthoracic catheters for transducing pulmonary artery and left atrial pressure. By using a combination of pressure measurements, oxygen saturation data, and green-dye curves, it is possible to obtain an indirect and relatively insensitive appraisal of the adequacy of a repair. None of these methods enables the surgical team to visually judge the degree of anatomic and functional normalcy achieved by the repair. Improved quantitative and qualitative methods for functional assessment of the heart and adequacy of surgical repair are needed.

With the advent of improved technology in echocardiography with Doppler color-flow imaging, preoperative diagnostic evaluation is able to provide detailed and precise delineation of even the most complex cardiac defects and their functional effect.[1] Recently, intraoperative transesophageal echocardiography (TEE) has been demonstrated to be an effective technique to assess cardiac function and anatomic defects in adult patients with valvular and ischemic heart disease.[2–5] The application of this same technology to the intraoperative evaluation of congenital heart defects would seem to be beneficial in providing surgeons and anesthesiologists with an additional means of assessing the quality of repair and functional results so that these patients can enjoy the best long-term outcome. Recently, the usefulness of intraoperative echocardiography during the repair of congenital heart lesions has been reported by several groups.[6–10]

This chapter summarizes the previously reported experience at the Duke Heart Center in using routine Doppler color-flow imaging both before and after cardiopulmonary bypass (CPB) for patients who were undergoing surgical correction of congenital heart defects.

TECHNIQUES AND METHODS

In general, intraoperative Doppler color-flow echocardiography includes the use of direct epicardial or transesophageal approaches during congenital heart surgery. In one study series, the majority of examinations were performed with epicardial techniques, although in some of the larger patients, TEE with Doppler color-flow imaging was also used.[10] The epicardial approach is useful in patients of all ages and sizes who undergo repair of congenital heart defects through a median sternotomy. The complex nature of many of these lesions favors the more versatile epicardial approach since it enables views of the anatomy from a variety of orientations, thus demonstrating each defect in exquisite detail. Using this approach, all major cardiac structures can be easily viewed, including all valves, chambers, septal structures, and great vessels. Not only does epicardial imaging require participation (and, therefore, focused concentration on the images) by the surgeon and the anesthesiologist, but the wide variety of view orientations enables superior interrogation of the numerous components of complex congenital defects and assessment of ventricular function and loading conditions.

For example, epicardial imaging provides a sensitive method to view the ventricular septum to identify the location of primary or residual defects. This approach can be applied at any time before, during, or after CPB, and epicardial imaging was not found to be disruptive to the flow of the surgical procedure.[10]

In these investigations, a Hewlett-Packard HP77020CF color-flow imaging system was used.[10] Transducer selection varied with patient size and the disease entity in question. Although the 5.0 MHz short focus transducer was used in the vast majority of cases, in certain cases a 2.5 MHz or 3.5 MHz transducer was also used. When deemed necessary, epicardial scans with a nonimaging 1.9 MHz continuous-wave Doppler probe were performed.

Before imaging, the transducer and cable are cleaned with a commercially available glutaraldehyde solution and left wrapped in a glutaraldehyde-soaked towel for at least 10 minutes. It is not necessary to gas sterilize the transducers that are to be used for epicardial images. Particular care should be taken to keep the liquid from entering the electrical contacts on the transducer assembly. The transducer is then wiped with sterile saline and taken to the patient's head where it is introduced into a sterile sheath that contains 20 ml of sterile ultrasound gel. The sheath is then secured to the surgical side of the ether screen, where it is available for use at any time during the operation (Fig. 8-1).

The transesophageal approach to intraoperative echocardiography with Doppler color-flow imaging has some application in children who are undergoing repair of congenital heart disease. The small size of many of these patients has limited the application of transesophageal techniques using the adult probe. Children who weigh greater than 10 to 12 kg are suitable candidates for using the adult probe. Since a considerable number of operations are performed in early infancy in small patients (less than 10 kg), the limitation of transesophageal probe size is a significant problem. Another limitation of the use of the transesophageal probe during congenital heart surgery is the restricted views from the esophagus. Esophageal probes are less maneuverable, especially in small patients, and, therefore, less capable of imaging certain aspects of anatomy.[11]

Although epicardial imaging has been preferred, transesophageal data acquisition has several attractive advantages. Transesophageal imaging can be performed continuously without requiring the surgeon to stop operating and, oftentimes, provides superior views of the mitral valve compared to those obtained from the epicardial approach. Another advantage is the continuous monitoring of ventricular function using the short-axis view.

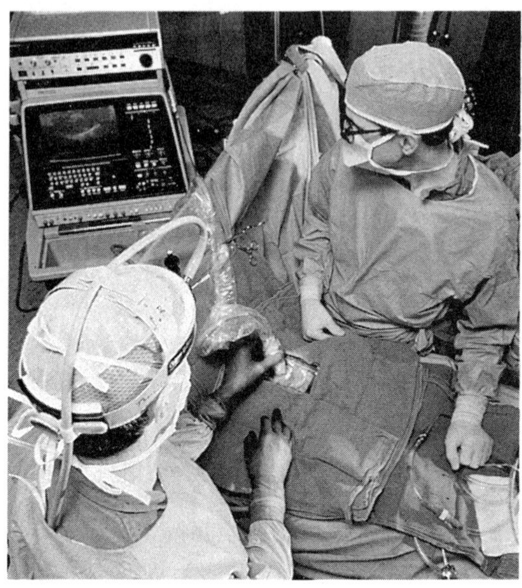

FIGURE 8-1. This intraoperative photograph shows how the epicardial transducer is readily available for use by the surgeon after insertion into a sterile sheath over the top of the anesthesia drapes. The color-flow monitor is easily positioned in a location where the surgeon and anesthesiologist can view the images in an on-line fashion as epicardial echocardiography is performed.

Technological advances, however, are providing TEE capabilities with smaller esophageal probes. One pediatric probe recently was evaluated in a few small infants who weighed less than 10 kg.[10] Because the smaller probe size incorporates fewer elements (32 as opposed to 64 in the conventional adult transesophageal probe), and has a smaller aperture, resolution of the two-dimensional image was considerably inferior. For example, difficulties were encountered in visualizing the endocardial-epicardial surfaces for the determination of ventricular wall motion. With advances in technology, clearer images for assessing anatomy with the pediatric probe should be forthcoming.

HISTORY OF INTRAOPERATIVE EPICARDIAL ECHOCARDIOGRAPHY

Johnson first reported the use of intraoperative epicardial echocardiography for the evaluation of results of mitral commissurotomy in 1972 using M-mode techniques.[12] Since then, multiple reports have been made of the use of epicardial echocardiography for a variety of specialized purposes using the two-dimensional technique.[13–17] Takamoto and colleagues first reported the use intraoperative echocardiography with color-flow mapping for a wide variety of clinical settings including repair of congenital heart defects.[18] Gussenhoven and colleagues recently reported the use of two-dimensional echocardiography in combination with contrast methods for intraoperative epicardial assessment in 195 patients with congenital heart disease.[6] In addition, Hagler and associates reported a preliminary series of 30 patients in which echocardiography with color-flow imaging was used in the operating room to assess repair of congenital heart lesions.[7] Recent reports suggest the potential advantages of color-flow imaging when used to evaluate repair of certain congenital cardiac defects.[6–10,19–21] No prospective reports are available, however, for a large number of such patients where two-dimensional pulsed- and continuous-wave Doppler and Doppler color-flow imaging were used routinely for the pre-CPB evaluation of the lesion and post-CPB assessment of surgical results.

CLINICAL EXPERIENCE WITH ECHOCARDIOGRAPHY USING DOPPLER COLOR-FLOW IMAGING AT DUKE

In an effort to understand the value of Doppler color-flow imaging in echocardiography, it was used prospectively both epicardially and transesophageally in 273 patients with congenital heart disease.[10] The intraoperative echocardiographic assessment using Doppler color-flow imaging was performed systematically in patients who were undergoing repair of congenital heart disease through a median sternotomy. Data were routinely acquired from the epicardial surface before initiation of CPB and again at the conclusion of the procedure, usually after the patient had been weaned from CPB. In some instances, additional data were obtained during periods of rewarming with the patient still on CPB. Studies included complete interrogation of all cardiac chambers and valves, including venous inflows and great vessel outflows. All data were recorded on high-fidelity videotape for later review.

In the study, all images were analyzed "on-line" in real-time, and decisions were made in each case on the basis of the echocardiographic data as well as any other relevant clinical observations available. All color-flow data were evaluated mutually and by consensus of the attending surgeon, anesthesiologist, and cardiologist present during the procedure. Medical and surgical management decisions were made on the basis of the Doppler information. Parasternal long-axis and four-chamber echocardiographic views with color-flow imaging were used to assess structural detail. A short-axis view of the heart was used to assess ventricular function. Ventricular dysfunction was defined as a change in wall motion (akinesia or dyskinesia) or the absence of systolic thickening on the post-CPB exam when compared to the baseline pre-CPB examination. The immediate impact of the echocardiographic findings on anesthetic and surgical management as well as information about residual structural and functional abnormalities after repair were recorded. Attempts were made to identify those patients whose surgical

TABLE 8-1. Intraoperative Echocardiography with Color-Flow Imaging for Congenital Heart Repair

Principal Diagnosis*	Number of Patients (Total = 273)
Tetralogy of Fallot	37
Ventricular septal defect	39
Atrial septal defect (primum + sinus venosus)	40
Atrioventricular septal defect	26
Valvular regurgitation	23
Congenital valvular aortic stenosis	15
Transposition of the great vessels	15
Univentricular heart	12
Pulmonary atresia	13
Tricuspid atresia/stenosis	9
Subvalvular aortic stenosis	9
Double outlet right ventricle	7
Aortic arch anomaly	7
Total anomalous pulmonary venous return	4
Coronary anomaly	4
Truncus arteriosus	2
Others	11

*Each patient counted only by major defect. Many patients had multiple defects.

(Data from Ungerleider RM, Greeley WJ, Sheikl KH et al: The use of intraoperative echo with Doppler color flow imaging to predict outcome following repair of congenital cardiac defects. Ann Surg 210:526, 1989)

and anesthetic management was influenced by intraoperative echocardiography because the findings were not apparent from the information available from the standard routine monitoring used. Follow-up short-term survival and reoperative data were collected in all patients.

To summarize the experience, echocardiography with Doppler color-flow imaging was used in 273 patients who were undergoing median sternotomy for correction of a variety of congenital cardiac defects. Diseases treated are listed by primary diagnosis in Table 8-1. Patients ranged in age from 1 day to 53 years (mean was 5.3 years), with 97 patients (37%) less than 1 year old and 152 patients (56%) less than 3 years old. The smallest patient weighed 1.8 kg. Data were collected from an epicardial transducer alone in 260 patients (96%), a transesophageal transducer alone in 4 patients (1%), and a combination of the two techniques in 9 patients (3%). The examination times are listed in Table 8-2 and illustrate the range that can be expected. The average study period for a complete examination was less than 4 minutes. Routine intraoperative color-flow echocardiography added an average of just less than 10 minutes to each case, most of this period as non-CPB time. In all patients, the quality of the intraoperative epicardial images were deemed superior to those obtained through the chest wall before surgery. Although contact of the transducer with the epicardial surface necessary to obtain good images would occasionally induce a few ectopic beats, the majority of the patients studied had no significant arrhythmias. No mediastinal infections occurred in this series.

In a systematic fashion, patients were routinely evaluated pre- and

TABLE 8-2. Number and Times of Examinations in 273 Patients

Examination	Minimum	Maximum	Mean	SD
Number of examinations	1	7	2.78	1.10
Duration of examinations (in minutes)				
Initial exam	0.18	12.00	4.00	1.89
Last exam	0.17	23.83	3.51	2.59
Total time/case	2.02	35.83	9.82	5.13
Average time/exam/case	0.76	17.91	3.64	1.73

SD = Standard deviation

(Data from Ungerleider RM: The use of intraoperative echocardiography with Doppler color flow imaging in the repair of congenital heart defects. Echocardiography 7:289, 1990)

post-CPB. Pre-CPB examinations disclosed the anatomy of each lesion in detail, far surpassing the preoperative transthoracic studies. In several cases, the pre-CPB exam demonstrated features of anatomy that had not been previously appreciated (Table 8-3). Although these findings were often judged to be insignificant because they had little impact on the operative plan, nevertheless, they provided a complete record of new anatomic information that became available to the surgeon at the time of operative repair.

An attempt was also made to assess whether the pre-CPB data were helpful in influencing the operative procedure. Data from the pre-CPB exam were evaluated as to whether they influenced anesthetic and surgical management. Echocardiography with color-flow imaging was judged helpful in planning when it contributed information that settled a preoperative uncertainty or provided data that influenced the conduct

TABLE 8-3. 63 Previously Unsuspected Details of Anatomy in 57 Patients (21%)

Details of Anatomy	Number
Anomalies of the Atrial or Ventricular Septum	
Atrial septal defect (none suspected)	12
Interatrial septal aneurysm	5
Multiple ventricular septal defects	5
Multiple atrial septal defects	5
Ventricular septal defect (non suspected)	3
Atrioventricular septal defect (complete)	1
Anomalies of Ventricular Inlet/Outlet	
Valvular anatomic or functional anomaly	6
Left or right ventricular outflow anomaly	3
Atrioventricular valve leaflet chordal anomaly	2
Functional flow anomaly (Tet spell)	2
Ventricular morphologic abnormality	2
Mitral systolic anterior motion	1
Anomalies of Venous Drainage	
Persistent left superior vena cava	6
Others	
Found normal anatomic structures thought absent	6
Patent ductus arteriosus	2
Residual shunt (Blalock-Taussig)	1
Located anomalous coronary different than cath	1

(Data from Ungerleider RM: The use of intraoperative echocardiography with Doppler color flow imaging in the repair of congenital heart defects. Echocardiography 7:289,1990)

of the case before or during the actual cardiac exploration (Table 8-4). In 127 patients (47%), the pre-CPB echocardiographic examination with color flow assisted anesthetic and surgical management. The ability to appreciate the specific anatomic and dynamic features of a defect immediately before institution of CPB was often felt to be quite beneficial by the surgical team. The most common reasons for affecting surgical management were changing the intraoperative surgical plan (69 patients) or guiding the intraoperative surgical approach (88 patients) (Fig. 8-2). The changes in anesthetic management initiated by pre-CPB color-flow imaging occurred in 10 patients (3.6%) and were usually of minor significance. Examples of color-flow imaging impact on anesthetic management include deepening of anesthetic level to reduce left ventricular outflow obstruction in a patient with unsuspected idiopathic hypertrophic subaortic stenosis physiology and hypotension, hyperventilation to reduce right ventricular distention in neonates with pulmonary hypertension (Fig. 8-3), and treatment of "tet" spells before they became clinically relevant (Color plate 5).

After completion of the operative procedure, color-flow echocardiography was used to evaluate the surgical repair and ventricular function. These data included both residual structural (surgical) abnormalities and residual abnormalities of ventricular function. Results were

TABLE 8-4. Impact of Echocardiography with Color-Flow Imaging on Case Planning

Impact		Number (Total)
Influence Operative Plan Prior to CPB		(69)
Change diagnosis	4	
Change operation	13	
Repair unsuspected lesion	15	
Influence approach to lesion	22	
Altered CPB plan	15	
Guide the Intraoperative Approach		(88)
Clarify valve and/or chordal commitments	25	
Indicate best manner for valve repair	9	
Identified precise location of defect	13	
Specify how to repair	41	
Alter Anesthesia Conduct Before CPB		(10)

CPB = Cardiopulmonary bypass

(Data from Ungerleider RM: The use of intraoperative echocardiography with Doppler color flow imaging in the repair of congenital heart defects. Echocardiography 7:289, 1990)

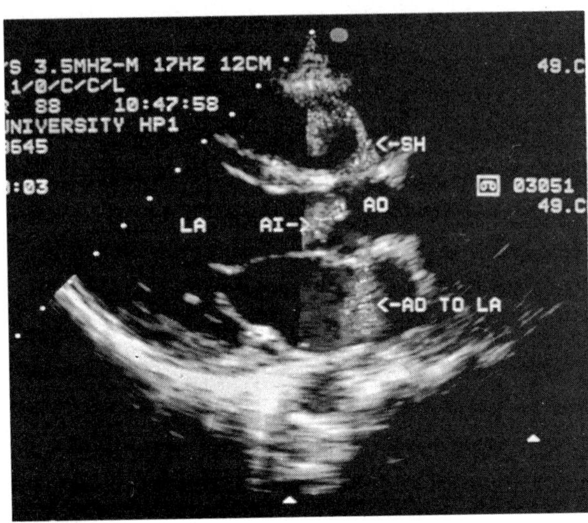

FIGURE 8-2. This prebypass epicardial examination is obtained from a 10-year-old who sustained a pellet gun wound to the heart. Although this child's pericardial tamponade was treated at another hospital, it was not noticed at that time (since echocardiography was not used during that procedure) that he has several intracardiac defects caused by the path that the pellet used to traverse the heart. Here the epicardial echocardiogram clearly delineates an aorta to right ventricle fistula *(SH)*, aortic insufficiency *(AI)*, and an aorta to left atrial fistula *(AO to LA)*. Knowledge of the precise location and nature of these defects just before institution of cardiopulmonary bypass facilitated proper identification and "echo-perfect" repair of this injury. *LA*, left artium; *AO*, aorta.

judged as "acceptable" (no significant residual structural defect) or "unacceptable" (residual structural defect of concern). These classes were based on echocardiographic Doppler color-flow images without regard to the patient's clinical condition. The patients with acceptable results had either "echo-perfect" repair (Fig. 8-4), without any evidence of persistent anatomic disturbance, or had minimal residual defects, which were felt to be quite insignificant given the well-known sensitivity of this technology (Fig. 8-5). If the post-CPB echo displayed residual shunt flow that was associated with pronounced turbulence and suggestive of more significant leak (Color plate 6), or if it displayed func-

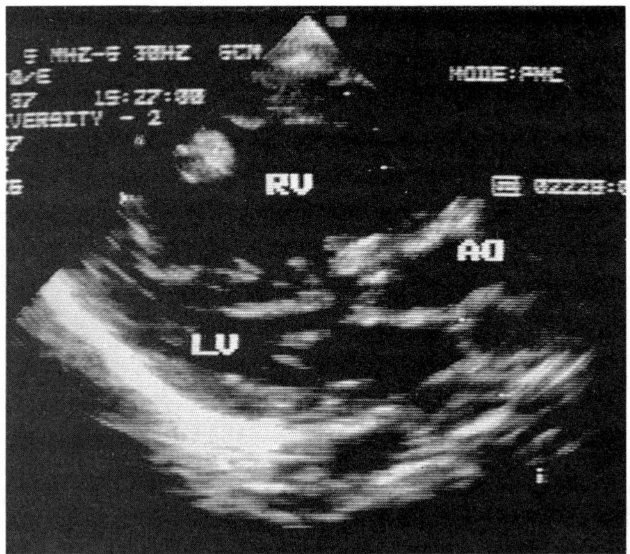

FIGURE 8-3. This long-axis image reveals displacement of the interventricular septum toward the left ventricle *(LV)* caused by pulmonary hypertension in an infant during the repair for interrupted aortic arch. This right ventricular *(RV)* dilatation was quickly and easily remedied by hyperventilation with 100% inspired oxygen. *AO,* aorta.

tion of a repaired valve that demonstrated persistent stenosis or regurgitation of moderate degree (Fig. 8-6), the repair was felt to be unacceptable. Any change in ventricular function from the pre-CPB status was also recorded. Records were kept to distinguish whether the dysfunction occurred in the right ventricle or left ventricle and whether these changes were global or located in a certain region, such as the ventricular septum. Changes in chamber size as well as changes in contractile patterns were noted. Finally, patients were also analyzed with respect to whether they left the operating room with any problem of concern compared to their preoperative exam and given the nature of their intended repair.

Patients were followed carefully for quality of outcome. To maintain as objective an appraisal as possible regarding outcome, definitive markers were chosen: reoperation for the same problem, at any time, or death. Death was classified as "surgical" (within 30 days of surgery) or "late" (beyond 30 days). Patients were recorded as having died, even

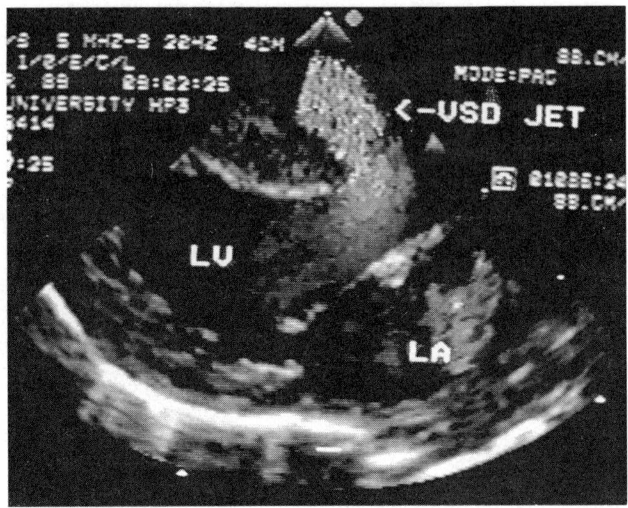

FIGURE 8-4A. A left-to-right shunt across a perimembranous ventricular septal defect *(VSD)* is easily imaged in this 1800-g infant.

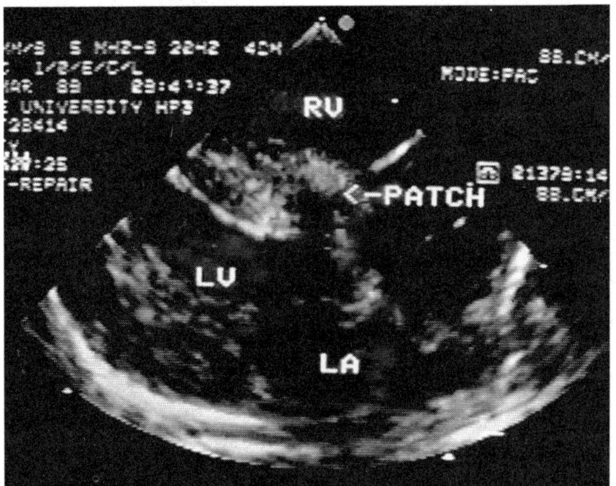

FIGURE 8-4B. After the repair, the *patch* can be seen to completely obliterate any residual shunt flow. This is an "echo-perfect" repair. *RV,* right ventricle; *LV,* left ventricle; *LA,* left atrium.

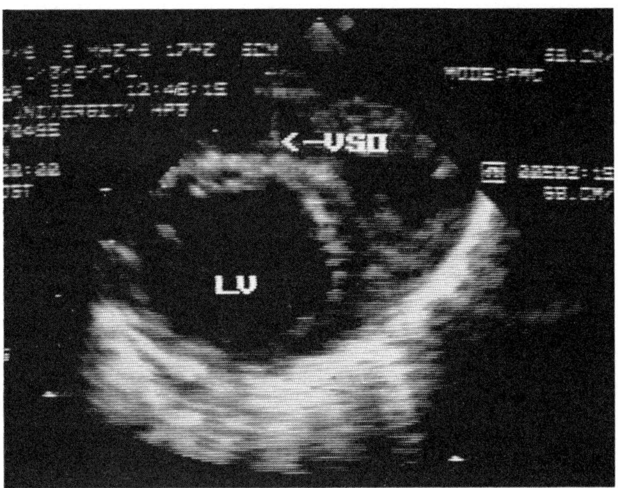

FIGURE 8-5. Short-axis view reveals a small residual ventricular septal defect *(VSD)* shunt at the inferior border of a patch. This finding is considered to be an insignificant residual defect and an "acceptable" result. *LV,* left ventricle.

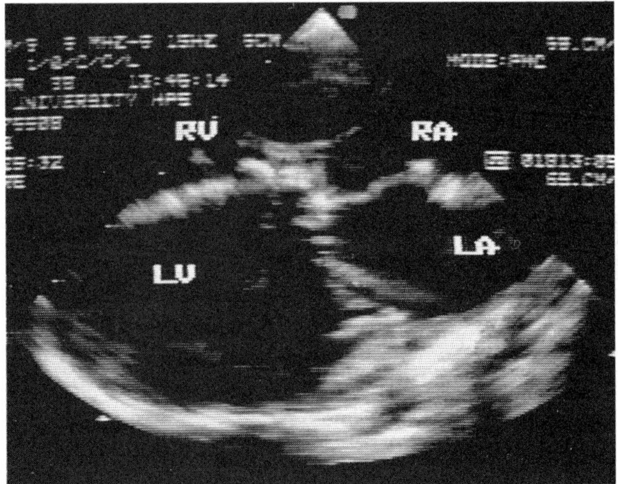

FIGURE 8-6. This image is obtained after repair of an atrioventricular canal defect in a 10-month-old infant. No residual ventricular septal defect shunt is seen but a moderate amount of residual mitral insufficiency is present. Although this finding did not require revision, and the patient has subsequently done well for more than 2 years of follow-up, this degree of mitral insufficiency is considered to represent a "residual defect of concern."

TABLE 8-5. Reason for Revision in 36 (13%) Patients

Reason	Redone	Acceptable Result
Clinical problem (Echo-Doppler confirms)	15	8
Echo-Doppler alone	21	18
Total	36	26

(Data from Ungerleider RM, Greeley WJ, Sheikh KH et al: The use of intraoperative echo with Doppler color flow imaging to predict outcome following repair of congenital cardiac defects. Ann Surg 210:526, 1989)

if they died from causes unrelated to their cardiac disease and regardless of whether or not they had been discharged from the hospital. Follow-up was performed for a range of 1 day to 2.1 years (mean was 1.02 plus or minus 0.58 years). No patients were lost to follow-up. Associations with specific residual structural and functional abnormalities and outcome were made.

Forty-seven patients (17%) presented echo findings of structural defects that were cause for concern after initial repair. In 36 of these patients, an attempt at revision was performed, and in 11 patients, no further surgery was performed. It is interesting to note that in the group of patients in whom revision was attempted, the data that led to the decision to reconstruct a portion of the repair was provided solely by color-flow echocardiography in 21 (58%) and from a combination of echo findings confirmed by clinical suspicions in 15 (42%). Eighteen (86%) of those patients whose repair was revised exclusively on the basis of echo information left the operating room with an acceptable

TABLE 8-6. Outcome Relating to Final Echo Results in 273 Patients

Residual Defect (Echo)	Number*	Acceptable Outcome	Reoperated	Surgical Death	Late Death
No residual defect	247 (90%)	210 (85%)	8 (3%)	24 (10%)	5 (2%)
Residual defect	24 (9%)	5 (21%)	10 (42%)	7 (29%)	2 (8%)
Cannot evaluate	2 (1%)	1 (50%)	0	1 (50%)	0

*Of entire series

$p < .006$ by Chi Square (compared to "No residual defect")

(Data from Ungerleider RM, Greeley WJ, Sheikl KH et al: The use of intraoperative echo with Doppler color flow imaging to predict outcome following repair of congenital cardiac defects. Ann Surg 210:526, 1989)

TABLE 8-7. **Impact of Residual Defect by Echocardiography**

Impact	Number	Acceptable Outcome	Reoperated	Surgical Death	Late Death
Repair before leaving operating room	26	22	1	2	1
No repair before leaving operating room	21	4*	10*	6	1

*p < .0125 by Chi Square (compared to "Repair before leaving operating room")

(Data from Ungerleider RM, Greeley WJ, Sheikh KH et al: The use of intraoperative echo with Doppler color flow imaging to predict outcome following repair of congenital cardiac defects. Ann Surg 210:526, 1989)

result by echocardiography. These 18 patients represent 7% of the entire series (Table 8-5).

Twenty-four patients in the overall series left the operating room with persistent residual defects as defined by echocardiography. Table 8-6 displays the impact of residual defects disclosed by color-flow imaging as they relate to the incidence of reoperation or death during the postoperative period. Table 8-7 separates the group of 47 patients who had initially unacceptable repairs (by echo color-flow examination) into two groups: those who left the operating room with an acceptable revision (26 patients) and those who left the operating room without revision (21 patients). This table documents the long-term outcome depending on how these relatively similar problems were dealt with before leaving the operating room.

In 68 (25%) patients, residual problems were of concern due to ventricular dysfunction. Ventricular dysfunction was defined as a change in wall motion (akinesia or dyskinesia) or absence of systolic thickening on the post-CPB echo-Doppler exam when compared to the baseline pre-CPB examination. The echocardiographic appearance of a new right ventricular wall motion abnormality (15 patients) carried a 33% mortality rate; a new left ventricular wall motion abnormality (40 patients) carried a 25% rate (Table 8-8). The presence of biventricular wall motion changes after repair (13 patients) carried a 69% rate of dying. Table 8-9 looks at outcome based on the presence of any post-CPB problem of concern as found by color-flow imaging (e.g., residual defects, ventricular dysfunction, disturbing anatomic or physiologic defect).

TABLE 8-8. Outcome Relating to Final Echo Results in 273 Patients

Ventricular Function (Echo)	Number*	Acceptable Outcome	Reoperated	Surgical Death	Late Death
No RV or LV problem	205 (75%)	180 (88%)	11 (5%)	8 (4%)	6
Only RV problem	15 (5%)	8 (54%)†	2 (13%)	5 (33%)†	0
Only LV problem	40 (15%)	24 (60%)†	5 (13%)	10 (25%)†	1 (2%)
Both RV and LV problems	13 (5%)	4 (31%)†	0	9 (69%)†	0

*Of entire series

†$p < .004$ by Chi Square (compared to "No RV or LV problems")

(Data from Ungerleider RM, Greeley WJ, Sheikh KH et al: The use of intraoperative echo with Doppler color flow imaging to predict outcome following repair of congenital cardiac defects. Ann Surg 210:526, 1989)

TABLE 8-9. Outcome Relating to Final Echo Results in 273 Patients

Any Residual Echo Concern	Number*	Acceptable Outcome	Reoperated	Surgical Death
No problems of concern	187 (68%)	170 (91%)	6 (3%)	7 (4%)
Problems of concern	86 (32%)	46 (54%)†	12 (14%)†	25 (29%)

*Of entire series

†$p < .0125$ by Chi Square (compared to "No problems of concern")

(Data from Ungerleider RM, Greeley WJ, Sheikl KH et al: The use of intraoperative echo with Doppler color flow imaging to predict outcome following repair of congenital cardiac defects. Ann Surg 210:526, 1989)

GENERAL DISCUSSION

The complexity of congenital heart defects, the diversity of surgical repairs, and the critical alterations in blood-flow patterns and function are challenges to the anesthesiologist and surgeon during operative management of patients with congenital heart disease. Current methods of intraoperative assessment are restricted to visual inspection of the heart and isolated pressure measurements, usually central venous pressure with occasional use of transthoracic catheters for pulmonary artery and left atrial pressure measurements. The recent development of a transesophageal echocardiographic probe has fostered a renewed interest in intraoperative echocardiography in adult cardiac patients.[2–5,15–17,22] However, this approach is not always useful in neonates, infants, and small children because of the large size of the probe and the restricted views from within the esophagus, which do not clearly assess the spectrum of cardiac anomalies in congenital heart disease. The majority of complex repairs are in small patients, and the transesophageal approach is not technically useful in assisting patient management. With the recent development of Doppler echocardiography with color-flow imaging, new information on cardiac function, structure, and blood-flow patterns in congenital heart disease has encouraged its use intraoperatively from the direct epicardial placement of the transducer in children. Data from the group presented here and from the work of other investigators demonstrate that intraoperative color-flow echocardiography can be quickly and efficiently performed during operations for the repair of congenital heart defects, even in small infants.

Echocardiography Doppler color-flow imaging improves intraoperative assessment of surgical repair of congenital heart defects and is an important adjunct to standard monitoring techniques in the assessment of the quality of repair of congenital heart defects. Its value in evaluating the quality of repair for congenital heart lesions is unparalleled by other methods. It is more sensitive than green-dye determinations in uncovering residual shunt defects (Fig. 8-7).[10] Although pressure measurements are useful in demonstrating and quantitating areas of residual stenosis, they do not demonstrate the etiology of the gradient; spectral analysis with Doppler, however, can not only predict the presence and degree of a residual stenosis, but, oftentimes, it demonstrates with unequivocal clarity the appropriate remedy. Oximetric data following a period of CPB is time-consuming, insensitive, and nonspecific and would seem to be the least reliable information available. Although these three kinds of assessments can provide complementing and useful information, a complete echo-Doppler evaluation takes an average of 3.6 minutes and provides a complete examination of the cardiac reconstruction and ventricular function. Defects such as insufficiency through a repaired valve may be identifiable only by this technology. The impressive sensitivity of this technology and the exceptional resolution that can be produced in images obtained directly from the epicardial surface and from the esophagus provide the surgeon and the anesthesiologist with an irreplaceable tool for evaluating the functional results of the surgical procedure.

Before CPB and operative repair, a complete echo-Doppler examination is able to demonstrate all of the features of anatomy and some features regarding cardiac function and loading conditions at a time

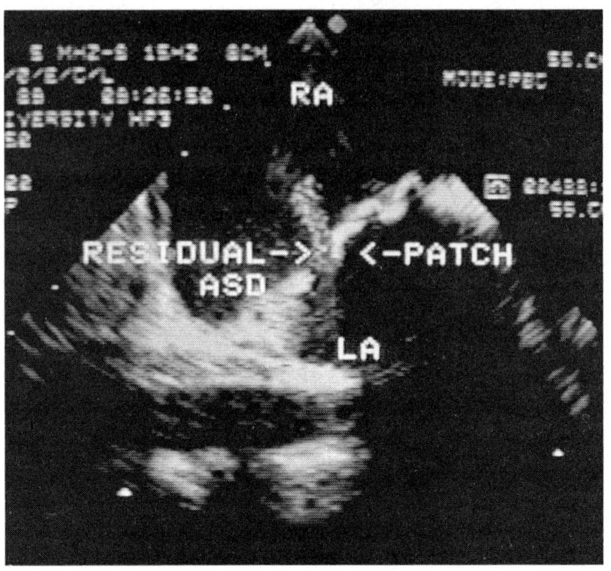

FIGURE 8-7A. This epicardial image reveals a *residual* left-to-right shunt at the edge of a *patch* placed to close an atrial septal defect *(ASD).* This is considered a "residual defect of concern." *RA,* right atrium; *LA,* left atrium.

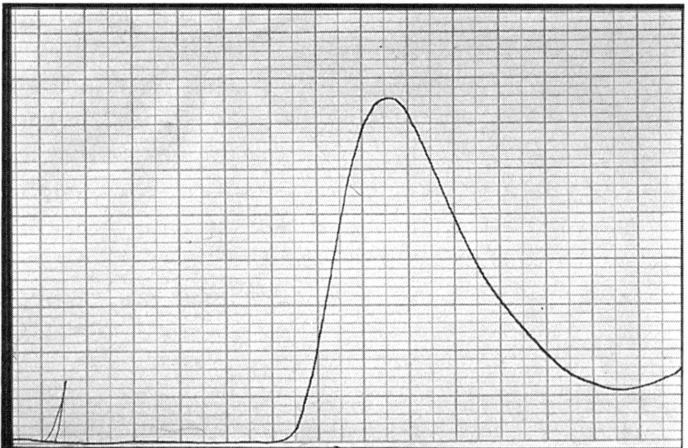

FIGURE 8-7B. The green dye-curve obtained after this patient was weaned from cardiopulmonary bypass shows that the residual echo-disclosed shunt is physiologically insignificant since this dye-curve demonstrates no left-to-right shunt.

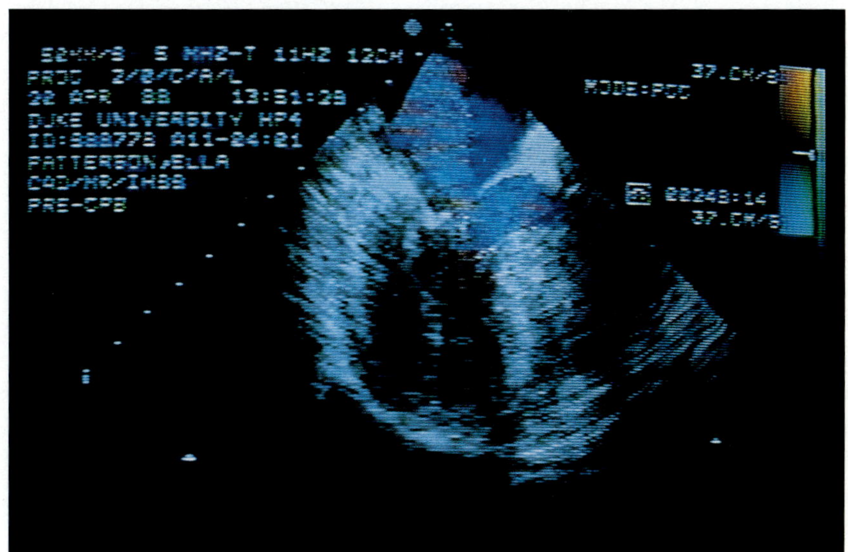

COLOR PLATE 1. Transesophageal echocardiography performed immediately after cardiopulmonary bypass identifies systolic turbulent color jets in the left ventricular outflow tract as well as in the left atrium, in a patient who has undergone mitral valve repair. Severe mitral regurgitation and outflow obstruction are present. This finding prompted revision of the mitral valve repair to placement of a mitral prosthesis, which corrected both the outflow obstruction as well as the mitral regurgitation.

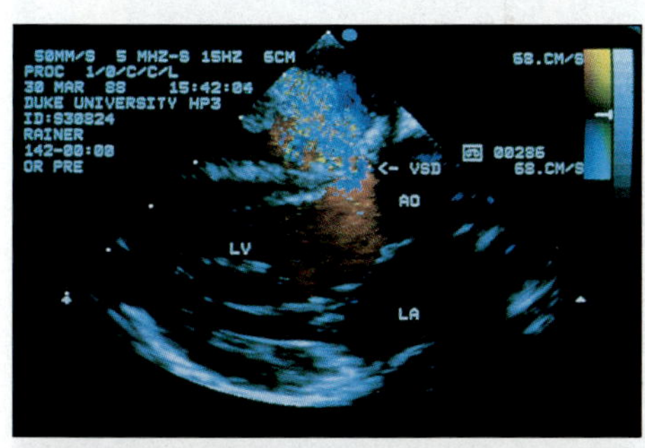

A

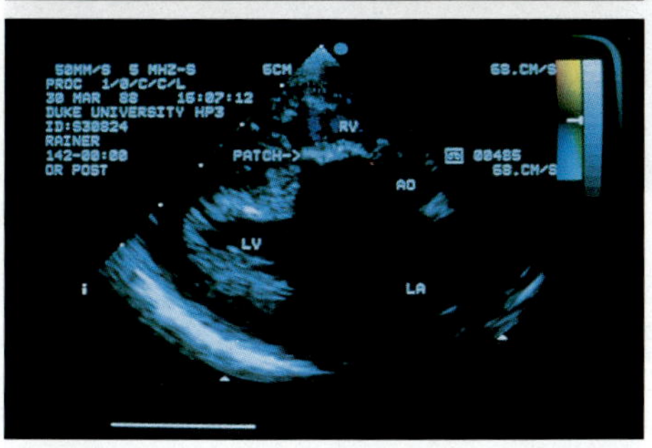

B

COLOR PLATE 2. *A,* Epicardial echocardiography before cardiopulmonary bypass shows a perimembranous ventricular septal defect with left to right shunting, indicated by the turbulent flow viewed in a parasternal long-axis image. *B,* After cardiopulmonary bypass, imaging indicates a successful patch placement without a residual leak identifiable by color-flow imaging.

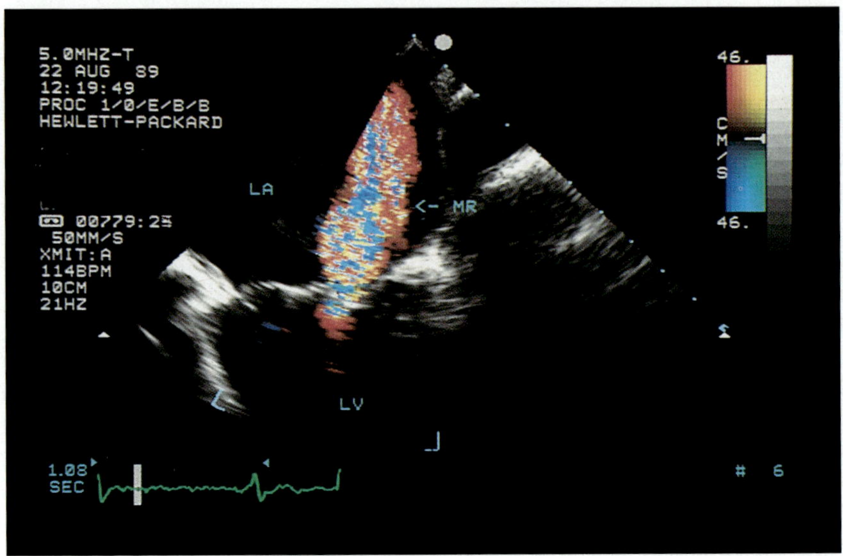

COLOR PLATE 3. In a long-axis transesophageal view of the mitral valve, it is easy to visualize the origin and extent of a mitral regurgitant jet. A variance color map has been used.

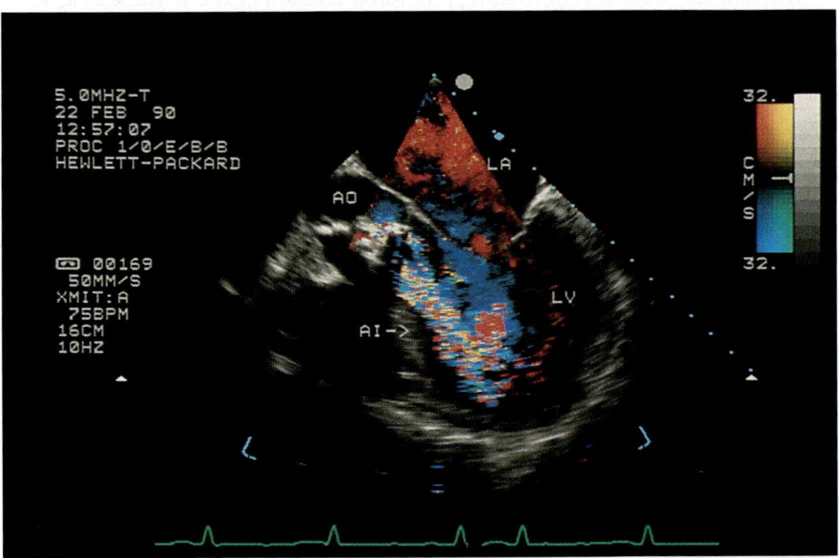

COLOR PLATE 4. In this example of aortic insufficiency, a bright jet can be seen in the left ventricular outflow tract well into the ventricle during diastole. This finding represents severe insufficiency.

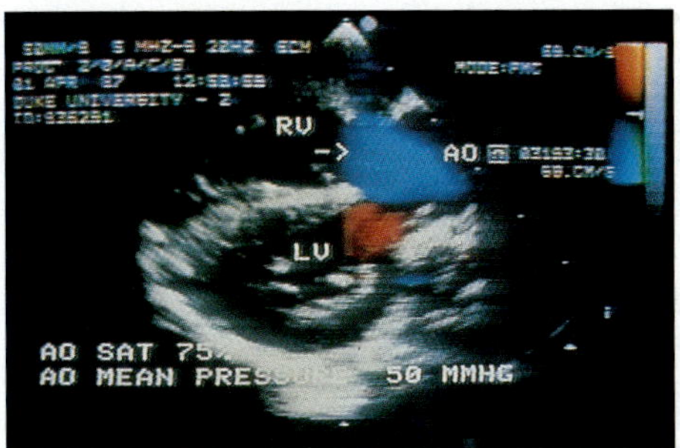

A

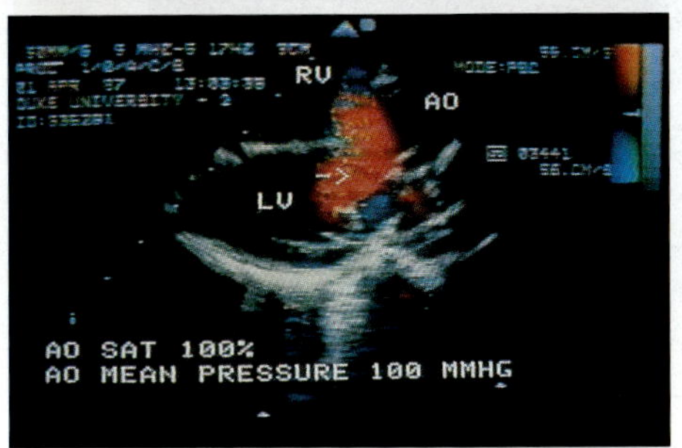

B

COLOR PLATE 5. *A,* Right-to-left shunting *(arrow)* across the ventricular septal defect in a patient with tetralogy of Fallot ("Tet spell") is easily remedied by raising the mean arterial pressure using phenylephrine. *B,* After institution of this therapy, the shunt is reversed and systemic arterial saturation rose from 75% to 100%. This patient underwent successful correction of his tetralogy defect. *(With permission from Greeley, et al. Anesthesia and Analgesia 68:815, 1989)*

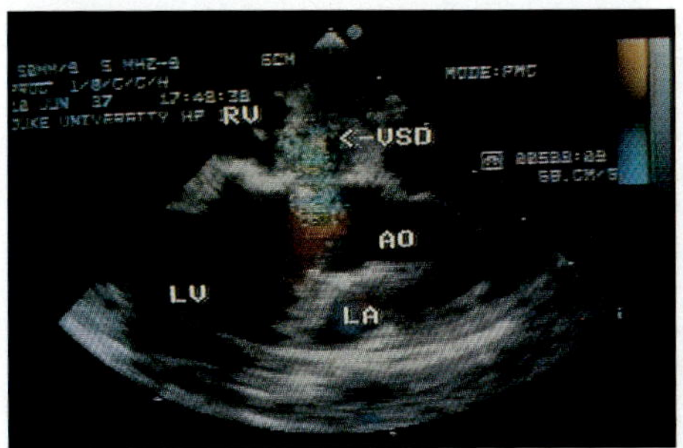

A

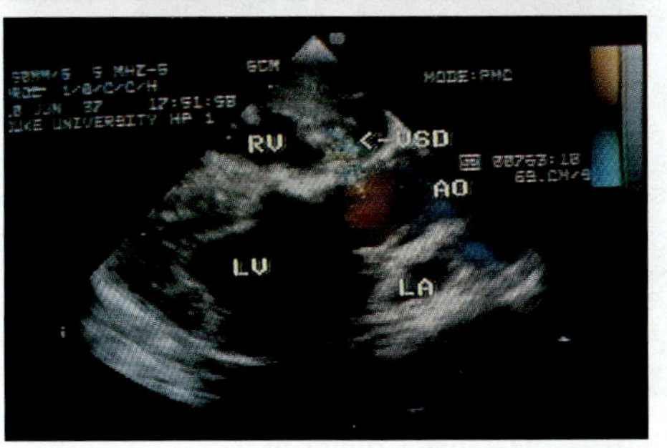

B

COLOR PLATE 6. *A,* This post-repair image is obtained from an infant after attempted correction of a complete AV canal defect. There is a large residual VSD shunt in the subaortic position. Despite the size of the shunt depicted by epicardial color-flow imaging, the patient was clinically well and had been weaned from cardiopulmonary bypass without difficulty. The infant was replaced on cardiopulmonary bypass and additional sutures were placed to close the defect. *B,* After revision, there is still a pronounced residual shunt though it has been reduced considerably in size. Nevertheless, this degree of residual shunt was considered moderate and "unacceptable."

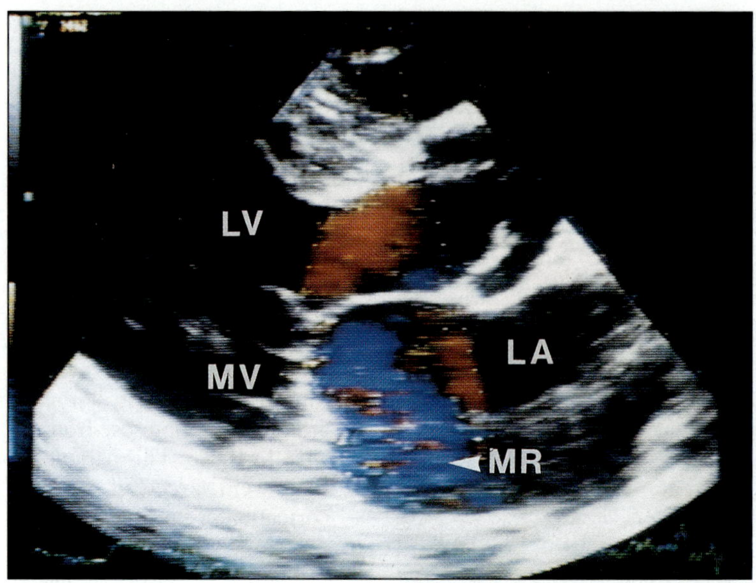

COLOR PLATE 7. Ischemic mitral regurgitation (*MR*) with normal leaflet morphology confirmed by visual inspection of the valve at surgery. Note the marked thinning of the inferior wall of the left ventricle. Epicardial parasternal-equivalent long-axis view of the left ventricle (*LV*), mitral valve (*MV*), and left atrium (*LA*) during systole.

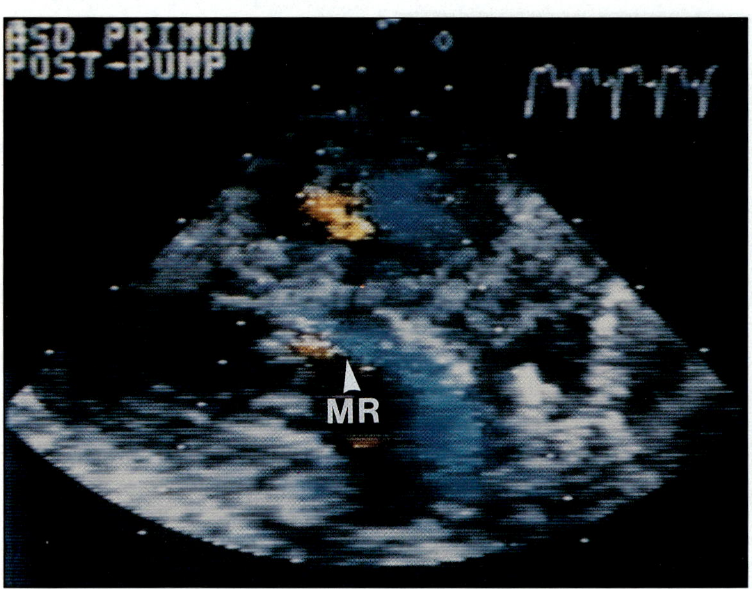

COLOR PLATE 8. Residual regurgitation *(MR)* after repair of a congenital cleft of the mitral valve. The cleft was not completely closed. Epicardial parasternal-equivalent long-axis view through the left ventricle, mitral valve, and left atrium.

when the surgeon is most interested with the plans for operative repair. Not infrequently, previously unappreciated details of anatomy are displayed so that they are considered by the surgeon as the design for the operative intervention is completed. In our experience, the pre-CPB echo-Doppler examination assisted anesthetic management and surgical planning in nearly half the cases in which it was performed. Assistance in specifying the surgical plan was the most common reason why it influenced pre-CPB management. Although the importance of these findings may vary for each institution, nevertheless, they allow the surgeon to begin the operative repair with a lucid mental image of the anatomy at hand. Likewise, the impact that these findings have on the conduct of the operation is also related in large part to the subjective appraisal of their importance by the surgeon and anesthesiologist and on the willingness of the surgical team to modify anesthetic and surgical management based on new information. For example, a surgeon who always opens the atrium to look for and close intra-atrial defects will not alter an operative plan if color-flow echocardiography uncovers a previously unappreciated atrial septal defect. However, a surgeon who does not routinely open the atrium to look for these defects may find this information quite useful. Likewise, an anesthesiologist who is interested in assessing the effect of intracardiac repair on ventricular function will find the pre-CPB examination of the short axis to be invaluable in obtaining a baseline evaluation, which can later be compared with post-CPB images for changes in function. Therefore, although the actual impact of pre-CPB imaging is arguable, it is unequivocal that this technology can demonstrate even the most complex anatomy and its physiologic alterations with exquisite detail, and baseline information that is generated may be useful during and after the repair.

Post-CPB examination with Doppler color-flow imaging is especially invaluable in assessing the quality of surgical repair and changes in ventricular function. Echocardiography with Doppler color-flow imaging is much more accurate in judging the adequacy of repair than the surgeon's opinion of the repair rendered before obtaining echo evaluation. Cases in which the surgeon was "satisfied" with the reconstruction, color-flow echocardiography disclosed a residual problem of some concern in 15%. However, even if the surgeon was dissatisfied with the reconstruction, echocardiography relieved those worries by disclosing an acceptable repair in 32% of those cases. Of particular interest is the importance of color-flow imaging in documenting concerns in the postrepair period. Eighteen patients in this series (7%) had immediate successful revision of their procedure based entirely on the information displayed by the color-flow images.[10] None of these patients demonstrated any suspicious clinical problems and without routine echo-Doppler color-flow imaging evaluation, most likely they would have left the operating room with a suboptimal repair. Echocardiography with color-flow imaging is an invaluable tool for assessing the quality of surgical repair in the immediate post-CPB period.

Epicardial and transesophageal echocardiography with color-flow imaging is also an extremely sensitive method for examining ventricular function. This particular assessment is performed simply by obtaining a short-axis view of the ventricles before and after repair. Contractility and chamber dimension of each ventricle can be compared to preoperative status. Although it is the goal of an efficient procedure to produce an accurate reconstruction without damaging cardiac function, 25% of the patients in our series had some alteration of ventricular function (determined by echocardiography) immediately post-CPB.[21] This alteration was not always clinically significant and did not always require treatment. Furthermore, the finding of decreased contractility was not necessarily an indication for inotropic therapy but had to be considered within the context of the physiology of the cardiac lesion. For example, increased right ventricular chamber size and decreased right ventricular contractility caused by pulmonary hypertension were sometimes best treated with hyperventilation. Left ventricular dysfunction from intramyocardial air was best treated by transient elevation of the blood pressure with phenylephrine, rather than with the use of inotropes (Fig. 8-8).[24] The usefulness of echo-Doppler color-flow imaging findings in directing intraoperative management has been previously described.[10] For evaluating ventricular function after repair of congenital heart defects, this technique serves as a sensitive method of identifying dysfunction and a means of assessing subsequent therapeutic interventions.

Little prospective information is available about identification of operative risk factors predictive of patient outcome for congenital heart surgery. Echocardiography with color-flow imaging may be useful in this regard. In a previous study, the post-CPB color-flow exam was important in evaluating the surgical repair for remaining problems of concern, and associations with short-term outcome were seen.[21] Ninety percent of the patients had no structural problems of concern after repair identified by echo-Doppler. The rate of reoperation at a later date was 3%, and the mortality rate was 10% in this group of patients. The remaining patients had residual problems of concern leaving the operating room because of structural defects. The presence of these residual structural abnormalities was associated with a 42% chance of reopera-

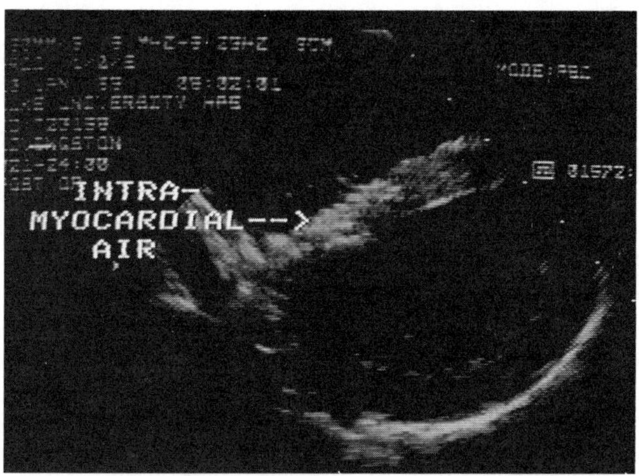

FIGURE 8-8A. After cardiopulmonary bypass, the short-axis view in this patient revealed a regional wall motion abnormality of the right ventricle, flattening of the interventricular septum, and evidence of ***intramyocardial air*** in the distribution of the right coronary artery. *(Greeley WJ, Kern FH, Ungerleider RM, Kisslo JA: Intramyocardial air causes right ventricular dysfunction after repair of a congenital heart defect. Anesthesiology 73:1042, 1990)*

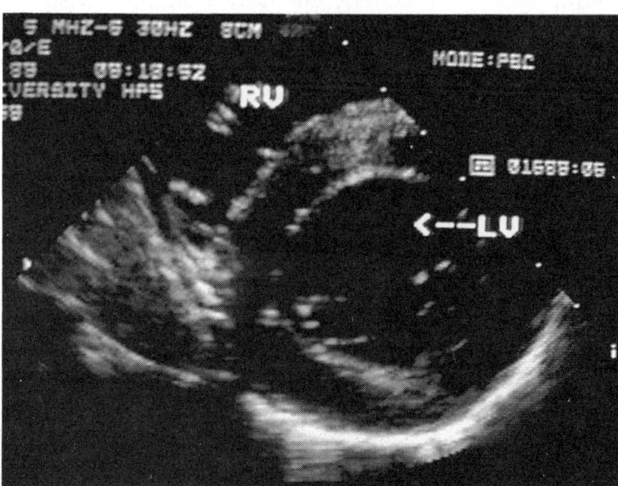

FIGURE 8-8B. After reperfusion on bypass and treatment with phenylephrine, repeat echo-Doppler demonstrated normal wall motion, normal position of the interventricular septem, and evacuation of intramyocardial air. ***RV,*** right ventricle; ***LV,*** left ventricle. *(Greeley WJ, Kern FH, Ungerleider RM, Kisslo JA: Intramyocardial air causes right ventricular dysfunction after repair of a congenital heart defect. Anesthesiology 73:1042, 1990)*

tion at a later date and a 29% mortality rate. Therefore, if the operation is completed and post-CPB echo-Doppler color-flow imaging fails to raise any concern with the result of the anatomic repair, the prognosis for a good outcome is better than 90%. However, if any concern is raised during the postrepair study, the likelihood of a good outcome is substantially decreased and may approach 50%.

Concerns about ventricular dysfunction identified by echocardiography with color-flow Doppler after repair were also predictive of outcome in our study.[21] The identification of a new right ventricular contraction abnormality as determined by a change in wall motion carried a 33% mortality rate. A new left ventricular wall motion abnormality carried a 25% rate. The presence of biventricular dysfunction after the repair yielded a 69% mortality rate. When no left or right ventricular changes were observed by echo-Doppler, the operative mortality rate was 4%. Whether intraoperative identification of ventricular dysfunction by the anesthesiologist and early therapeutic interventions will improve outcome remains to be determined. Nonetheless, early identification certainly assists the anesthesiologist and surgeon in the intraoperative management of these patients.

The absence of residual structural and functional abnormalities on echocardiography with Doppler color-flow imaging is associated with a low reoperative rate and a high survival rate.[21] Ventricular dysfunction and residual structural defects identified by echo-Doppler are associated with an increased chance of reoperation and a high mortality rate. All data that led to the generation of these rates were provided prospectively, in the operating room at the time of surgery.[10,21] This fact means that the surgeon and anesthesiologist who become familiar with the interpretation of echo-Doppler have the ability to quickly generate predictive information about the quality of the operative repair before the patient leaves the operating suite. Furthermore, the nature of this information guides a direct and efficient modification of the procedure when appropriate to mend a residual defect or to revise a technical inaccuracy or to initiate early therapeutic interventions for ventricular dysfunction.

During the repair of complex congenital heart defects, the anesthesiologist and surgeon are occasionally confronted with a patient who is difficult to wean from CPB. Under these circumstances, identification of the problem, that is, residual structural defect that requires rerepair vs. a functional abnormality that requires pharmacologic support, is difficult to assess. Neonates, infants, and children with minimal cardiac reserve may not tolerate hemodynamic instability for long periods of time under these conditions. Interventions must be made quickly and rationally based on available clinical information. The subjective experience of the surgeon and the anesthesiologist often becomes the primary determinant for altering support or assessing the adequacy of repair. Echo-Doppler provides an additional method for rapidly diagnosing functional and structural abnormalities that assists the anesthesiologist and surgeon in selecting the appropriate medical or surgical therapy.[10] For the anesthesiologist, echo-Doppler identification of intramyocardial air or a new wall motion abnormality may direct specific pharmacologic interventions and provide a means of assessing the results of these interventions. For the surgeon, identification of residual anatomic defects may lead to immediate reinstitution of CPB, correction of the defect, and subsequent weaning from bypass.

Although the nature of the data appears to be subjective, a surgical team can learn to interpret their intraoperative echocardiographic data with respect to repair of congenital cardiac defects. The information provided by echocardiography with color-flow Doppler shortened the learning curve by teaching the surgical team the location of problems and gave immediate positive reinforcement to techniques that avoided these problems in subsequent patients.

TRAINING REQUIREMENTS

With the development of Doppler color-flow imaging, an interest in intraoperative echocardiography during the repair of congenital heart defects has been fostered. Echocardiographic techniques are becoming more widely used in the operating room to define normal and abnormal cardiac anatomy, evaluate cardiac chamber sizes and dynamics, and assess valvular disease, both before and after repair. Surgeons and anesthesiologists can be trained to become more expert in the conduct and interpretation of the Doppler color-flow examinations to assure high-quality data. Anesthetic and surgical judgment and skills are acquired over time and the same applies to echocardiography. A long, intensive cooperative effort between experienced cardiologists with surgeons or anesthesiologists less experienced in ultrasound methods is required.

Intraoperative echocardiographic evaluation of the patient with congenital heart disease involves the use of several related ultrasonic techniques that require an understanding of the underlying principles, instrumentation, application advantages, and limitations. The extent of optimal physician training in echocardiography to attain the technical expertise in these diagnostic techniques has not been firmly established. Proper development of these skills requires training under the guidance of an experienced echocardiographer. The American Society of Echocardiography Committee for Physician Training in Echocardiography has identified three levels of training (introductory, intermediate, and advanced) in echocardiography and recommends that physicians obtain the equivalent levels of expertise appropriate to their needs.[23] Specialized expertise is needed for the physician (cardiologist, surgeon, and anesthesiologist) who uses intraoperative echocardiography during the repair of complex congenital heart disease. Based on our experience we found two levels of training necessary. Identification of ventricular wall motion abnormalities and function in the short-axis view using either an epicardial or transesophageal approach requires approximately 3 months of consistent training and includes the application of 100 to 200 examinations intraoperatively. Identification of wall motion abnormalities have been shown to be relatively easy to learn. The second level, that is, the ability to generate diagnostic information and render an interpretation, requires significantly more experience and expertise. It is difficult to specify the length of training necessary for a physician to achieve this level of competence. The ability to evaluate complex congenital heart defects seems to require approximately 1 year of continuous training and at least 300 patient studies in the operating room before sufficient expertise is developed to make independent diagnostic judgments and to use results to determine patient management. Since the decision to reoperate and place the patient back on bypass is of critical magnitude, application of echocardiographic techniques in this regard becomes very important.

These guidelines represent only a general framework. Ideally, the best approach to intraoperative echocardiographic analysis requires a team of competent physicians working together. This team should consist of an experienced physician-echocardiographer, surgeon, and anesthesiologist well practiced in the discipline. Echocardiographic information must be taken in the context of overall patient management, which includes surgical judgment and interpretation of the standard monitoring modalities used by the anesthesiologist when determining a clinical decision.

This effort requires a large capital investment. It may be argued that the capital equipment requisite for the performance of such studies is excessive. Data from this past study indicate that, if the ultrasound system was left in the room for the entire procedure, it would be in use only 6% of the time. Several methods are available to reduce such overhead. Given the safety of using a sterile sheath, expensive transducers do not have to be gas sterilized, thus making them available for clinical use when not in the operating room. Leaving the transducer in the sterile field during longer cases but taking the system out of the room for other clinical purposes also helps to reduce the overhead. The savings in operating room time and the possible prevention of reoperation due to less than optimal results justifies the remaining cost. Furthermore, routine use of intraoperative echocardiography with Doppler color-flow imaging results in familiarity with its application and provides the surgeon and anesthesiologist with an additional technique to evaluate the quality of operative results.

CONCLUSIONS

Intraoperative echocardiography with Doppler color-flow imaging is helpful to the anesthesiologist and surgeon as an adjunctive monitoring technique during the repair of complex congenital heart defects, especially in the young patient. For this purpose, it may be performed from either the epicardial or transesophageal approach, although the latter has significant limitations due to patient size and restrictive imaging views. Post-repair echocardiographic examination is able to assess adequacy of surgical repair as well as identify functional abnormalities of the ventricle. Further, identification of residual abnormalities is predictive in assessing surgical outcome. While no method can replace anesthetic and surgical judgment, experience, or skill, echocardiography with color-flow imaging is, nevertheless, a valuable addition for the immediate assessment of operative results. The ability of this method to predict operative outcome may, in the future, lead to new approaches in the repair or management of complex congenital heart defects.

References

1. Sahn DJ: Real-time two-dimensional Doppler echocardiographic flow mapping. Circulation 71:849, 1985
2. de Bruijn NP, Clements FM, Kisslo JA: Intraoperative transesophageal color flow mapping: Initial experience. Anesth Analg 66:386, 1987
3. Cahalan MK, Litt L, Botvinick EH, Schiller NB: Advances in noninvasive cardiovascular imaging: Implications for the anesthesiologist. Anesthesiology 66:356, 1987
4. Smith JS, Cahalan MK, Benefiel DJ et al: Intraoperative detection of myocardial ischemia by echocardiography. Circulation 72:1015, 1985

5. Matsumoto M, Oka Y, Strom J et al: Application of transesophageal echocardiography to continuous intraoperative monitoring of left ventricular performance. Am J Cardiol 46:95, 1980
6. Gussenhoven EJ, van Herwerden LA, Roelandt J, Ligtvoet KM, Bos E, Witsenburg I: Intraoperative two-dimensional echocardiography in congenital heart disease. J Am Coll Cardiol 9:565, 1987
7. Hagler DJ, Tajik AJ, Seward JB, Schaff HV, Danielson GK, Puga FJ: Intraoperative two-dimensional Doppler echocardiography: A preliminary study for congenital heart disease. J Thorac Cardiovasc Surg 5:516, 1988
8. Greeley WJ, Stanley TE, Ungerleider RM, Kisslo JA: Intraoperative hypoxemic spells in tetralogy of Fallot: An echocardiographic analysis of diagnosis and treatment. Anesth Analg 68:815, 1989
9. Ungerleider RM, Kisslo JA, Greeley WJ et al: Intraoperative prebypass and postbypass epicardial color flow imaging in the repair of atrioventricular septal defects. J Thorac Cardiovasc Surg 98:90, 1989
10. Ungerleider RM, Greeley WJ, Sheikh KH et al: Routine use of intraoperative, epicardial echo and Doppler color flow imaging to guide and evaluate repair of congenital heart lesions: A prospective study. J Thorac Cardiovasc Surg 100:287, 1990
11. Bolger A, Czer LSC, Friedman A et al: Intraoperative transesophageal color Doppler imaging: Advantages and limitations (abstr). J Am Coll Cardiol 11:217, 1988
12. Johnson ML, Holmes JH, Spangler RD, Patton BC: Usefulness of echocardiography in patients undergoing mitral valve surgery. J Thorac Cardiovasc Surg 64:922, 1972
13. Harrison LH, Kisslo JA, Sabiston DC: Extraction of intramyocardial foreign body utilizing operative ultrasonography. J Thorac Cardiovasc Surg 82:345, 1981
14. Spotnitz HM, Malm JR: Two-dimensional ultrasound and cardiac operations. J Thorac Cardiovasc Surg 83:43, 1982
15. Mindich BP, Goldman ME, Fuster V, Burgess N, Litwak R: Improved intraoperative evaluation of mitral valve operations utilizing two-dimensional contrast echocardiography. J Thorac Cardiovasc Surg 90:112, 1985
16. Maurer G, Czer LSC, Chaux A et al: Intraoperative Doppler color flow mapping for assessment of valve repair for mitral regurgitation. Am J Cardiol 60:333, 1987
17. Czer LSC, Maurer G, Bolger AF: Intraoperative evaluation of mitral regurgitation by Doppler color flow mapping. Circulation 76:108, 1987
18. Takamoto S, Kyo S, Adachi H et al: Intraoperative color flow mapping by real-time two-dimensional Doppler echocardiography for evaluation of valvular and congenital heart disease and vascular disease. J Thorac Cardiovasc Surg 90:802, 1985
19. Sutherland G, Smyllie J, Roelandt J: Color flow imaging as intraoperative angiography in ventricular septal defects: Advantages and pitfalls? J Am Coll Cardiol 13:75A, 1989
20. Ungerleider RM: The use of intraoperative echocardiography with Doppler color flow imaging in the repair of congenital heart defects. Echocardiography 7:289, 1990
21. Ungerleider RM, Greeley WJ, Sheikh KH et al: The use of intraoperative echo with Doppler color flow imaging to predict outcome following repair of congenital cardiac defects. Ann Surg 210:526, 1989

22. Stewart WJ, Currie PJ, Lytle BW, Gill CC, Cosgrove DM: The role of intraoperative echocardiography during cardiac valvular surgery (abstr). J Am Coll Cardiol 11:217, 1988
23. Pearlman AS, Gardin JM, Martin RP et al: Guidelines for optimal physician training in echocardiography: Recommendations of American Society of Echocardiography Committee for Physician Training in Echocardiography. Am J Cardiol 60:158, 1987
24. Greeley WJ, Kern FH, Ungerleider RM, Kisslo JA: Intramyocardial air causes right ventricular dysfunction after repair of a congenital heart defect. Anesthesiology 73:1042, 1990

Lawrence S. C. Czer
Gerald Maurer

9 Epicardial Echocardiography and Doppler Color-Flow Mapping in the Adult Patient

Epicardial echocardiography is a versatile technique that provides a near continuum of images of the heart because of the wide variety of transducer positions and orientations available. All of the cardiac valves and chambers, as well as the proximal aorta and pulmonary artery, can be imaged from the epicardial approach. Coronary bypass grafts and coronary arteries can also be imaged.

Suitable candidates for epicardial Doppler color-flow imaging include patients with suspected valvular regurgitation, patients who are undergoing a valve repair procedure, those with an ischemic ventricular septal defect or other intracardiac shunt, and patients who are undergoing intraoperative remodeling procedures such as balloon or laser angioplasty of the coronary arteries or bypass grafts. Epicardial imaging may also be appropriate when transesophageal imaging is contraindicated due to esophageal disease (stricture, erosion, neoplasm) or an increased risk of mucosal bleeding (varices, severe coagulopathy).

TECHNIQUE

Imaging

Epicardial echocardiographic imaging is usually performed with a 3.5 or 5.0 MHz transducer. Greater resolution is provided by the higher frequency transducer, but it has less penetrance, so that very large hearts may not be optimally imaged; in addition, color Doppler aliasing occurs at lower velocities because the Nyquist limit is less. With very small cardiac structures, even higher frequency transducers are used because of the requirement for increased resolution. Coronary arteries and bypass grafts can be imaged with a 12.5 MHz mechanical sector scanner. (Surgiscan, BioSound Corporation, Indianapolis, Indiana). A prototype 7.5 MHz transducer with color Doppler imaging capability has also been utilized at some centers, but is not widely available.

The transducer is covered with a sterile plastic sheet or sleeve after placing sonolucent gel on the imaging surface of the transducer to provide acoustic coupling. The entire length of the cord that leads from the transducer to the color Doppler machine is also covered with the sterile plastic sheet. Before placing the transducer assembly on the epicardial surface of the heart, the epicardium is moistened with sterile saline solution to ensure an adequate acoustic interface. Care must be observed to avoid folds and irregularities of the plastic covering of the imaging surface of the transducer so that epicardial abrasions do not occur and image quality is not compromised.

From the midanterior surface of the right ventricle, the heart can be imaged in parasternal-equivalent long- and short-axis views (Figs. 9-1 and 9-2). In long-axis with the button on the transducer oriented toward the ascending aorta, the left atrium, mitral valve, left ventricle, left ventricular outflow tract, aortic valve, and aorta are imaged. Rotating the transducer 90 degrees clockwise and tilting the tip upward, the right atrium, tricuspid valve, right ventricle, infundibulum, pulmonic valve, proximal pulmonary artery, left atrium, and ascending aorta are

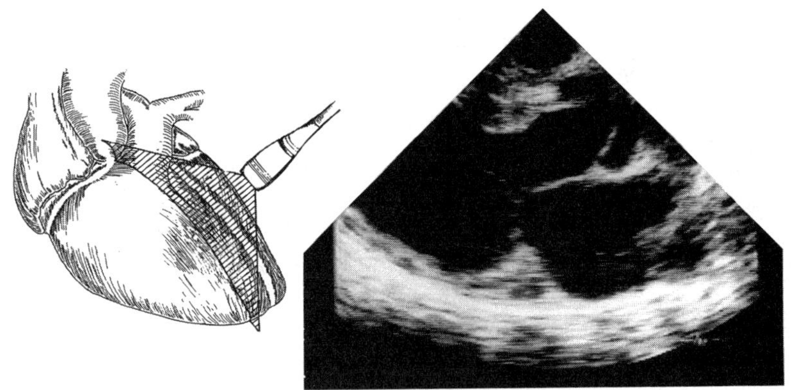

FIGURE 9-1. Imaging plane for parasternal-equivalent long-axis view *(left)* and corresponding two-dimensional echocardiographic image *(right)*.

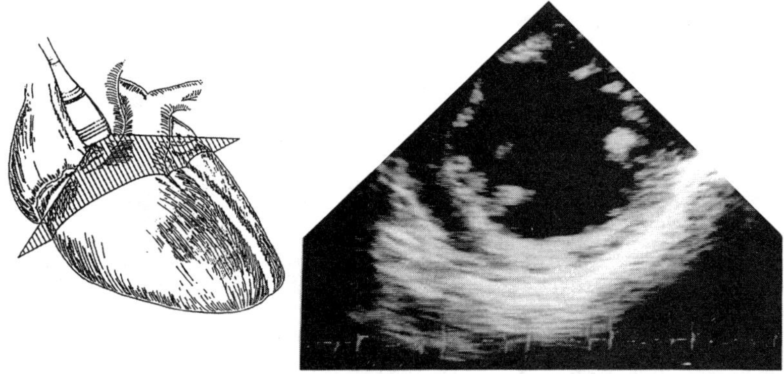

FIGURE 9-2. Imaging plane for parasternal-equivalent short-axis view at the level of the papillary muscles *(left)* and corresponding two-dimensional echocardiographic image *(right).*

imaged in short axis. Tilting the transducer tip downward, a succession of short-axis views of the left atrium, aortic valve, mitral valve, and left ventricle can be obtained. Moving the transducer assembly inferiorly toward the diaphragmatic surface of the right ventricle and tilting the transducer tip upward with the button oriented toward the right atrium, a subxiphoid-equivalent four-chamber long-axis view of the heart is obtained (Fig. 9-3). This view is particularly useful for imaging the right

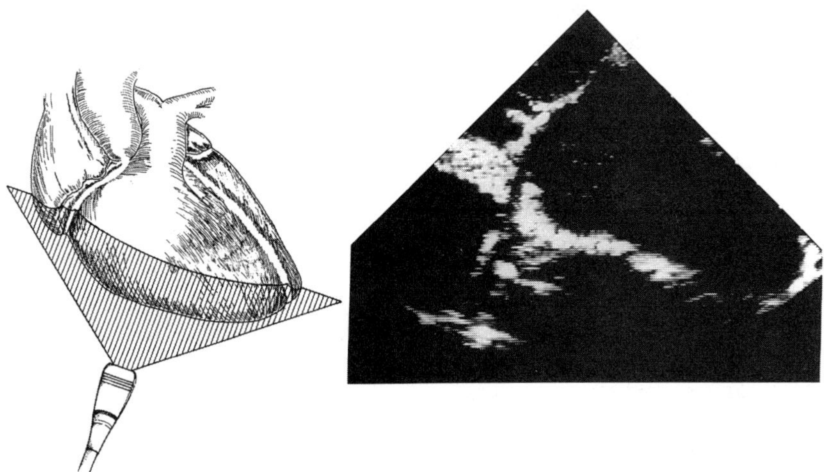

FIGURE 9-3. Imaging plane for subxiphoid-equivalent four-chamber view *(left)* and corresponding echocardiographic image *(right).*

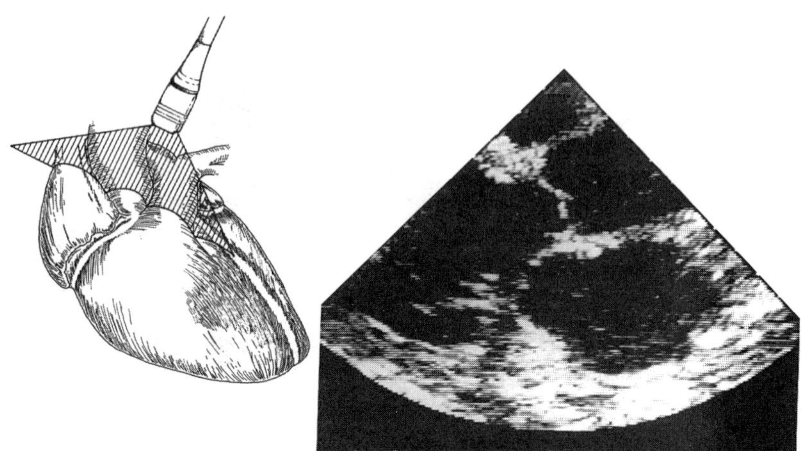

FIGURE 9-4. Imaging plane for aorto-pulmonary sulcus view *(left)* and corresponding echocardiographic image *(right)*.

atrium, tricuspid valve, and right ventricle. Short-axis views may be obtained by rotating the transducer 90 degrees clockwise. Finally, by placing the transducer on either side of the aorta (in the aorto-pulmonary or aorto-superior venae caval sulci), long-axis views of the ascending aorta, aortic valve, mitral valve, and left atrium can be obtained (Fig. 9-4). This view has been useful for examining flow across the aortic valve and in the ascending aorta, as well as for eccentric jets in the left atrium. It has also been useful in reoperated patients with adhesive pericarditis and in patients with extensive pericardial fat because epicardial views obtained from the midright ventricle often demonstrate poor image quality in these patients.

During imaging, the electrocardiogram, right atrial, pulmonary arterial, pulmonary capillary wedge, and systemic arterial pressures are recorded. For assessment of mitral or tricuspid regurgitation, intravenous fluids or phenylephrine are administered when needed to attain preload and afterload conditions comparable to those at catheterization or at the preoperative resting state.[1,2] Imaging and hemodynamic measurements are repeated in a similar manner after cardiopulmonary bypass and rewarming, taking care to match preload and afterload conditions as closely as possible to the prepump state.

Mitral or tricuspid regurgitation is graded semiquantitatively on a scale of 0 to 4+, according to the maximal systolic length of the regurgitant jet in relation to the atrium: 1+ is assigned if the jet extends immediately behind the valve, 2+ if it extends up to one third of the length of the atrium, 3+ if up to two-thirds, and 4+ if more than two-thirds into the atrium.[1,2] Alternatively, the grading system of Helmcke and associates may be used, in which the maximal area of the regurgitant jet is compared with the atrial area.[3,4] In patients with mitral regurgitation, a ratio of less than 20% corresponds to mild regurgitation, 20% to 40% to moderate, and greater than 40% to severe regurgitation.[3] In patients with tricuspid regurgitation, a ratio greater than 34% indicates severe regurgitation.[4]

Color Doppler gain is adjusted to a level just below excessive random noise (5% of pixels). Low velocity swirling flows that are separate from a primary regurgitant jet are usually ignored in the grading of regurgitation; the ability to image these low-velocity flows depends on the pulse repetition frequency, frame rate, velocity threshold, depth, sector width, and gain setting. Studies are obtained at frame rates of 7.5 to 30 per second and usually at middle pulse repetition frequencies. Images are recorded on ½-inch videotape, and hemodynamic pressures on a strip chart recorder.

Safety Considerations

Electrical current consumption ranges from 7 to 15 A for most color Doppler systems. To prevent potentially catastrophic circuit overload or power failure, color Doppler equipment should be connected to electrical circuits that do not supply other operating room equipment. Hospital-grade plugs with appropriate grounding must be used. Leakage currents should be minimal. Color Doppler systems should be used cautiously in the presence of flammable agents.

To maintain sterility, the probe drape or sleeve should be leakproof; its condition should be checked before and after each procedure. Sterilization of the ultrasound transducer by ethylene oxide gas has a corrosive effect that may damage the transducer after repeated applications; therefore, the use of gas sterilization generally is not recommended.

ASSESSMENT OF MITRAL OR TRICUSPID REGURGITATION

Importance of Afterload

Changes in afterload conditions may substantially influence the severity of mitral or tricuspid regurgitation and its grading by color Doppler techniques. In 22 patients with mitral regurgitation, a planimetered area, circumference, length, and width of the left atrium and the maximal regurgitant jet from color Doppler still frames in the parasternal-equivalent long-axis view. Images and hemodynamics were recorded before and after phenylephrine infusion (mean dose, 150 μg; range 50–300). Phenylephrine was administered to adjust the systolic pressure to a level comparable to that obtained at preoperative cardiac catheterization (Table 9-1). It should be noted that the initial baseline pressures were significantly lower than those obtained after phenylephrine infusion.

After phenylephrine infusion, the absolute jet dimensions as well as the jet in relation to the left atrial size (jet to left atrial ratio) all increased significantly (Table 9-2). Furthermore, the increase in systolic pressure consistently produced an increase in jet area in absolute and relative terms (Fig. 9-5). Similar findings were observed for the other jet dimensions (length, width, and circumference). Thus, mitral regurgitant jet size was substantially affected by afterload as measured by the systolic pressure. By implication, care must be exercised to match intraoperative systolic pressure to baseline or fixed reference levels when evaluating mitral regurgitation.

It should be noted, however, that the change in jet area could not be predicted on the basis of the change in systolic pressure alone (Fig. 9-6). In fact, many other physiologic variables may also influence regurgitant jet size, including the left atrial pressure, the atrial size and compliance, pulmonary venous compliance, regurgitant orifice size, and papillary muscle function. Many technical factors may influence color Doppler jet size measurement, such as the gain setting, the pulse repetition frequency, imaging of the low velocity swirling flows, differentiation of regurgitation from displacement flow, complexities in jet

TABLE 9-1. Intraoperative Hemodynamics Before and After Phenylephrine and Comparison with Values at Preoperative Cardiac Catheterization*

Hemodynamic Variable	Cardiac Catheterization	Intraoperative	
		Baseline	*Phenylephrine*
Systolic pressure	134 ± 27	108 ± 14	137 ± 17†
PCW mean	20 ± 8	11 ± 5	21 ± 11†
PCW V wave	26 ± 13	13 ± 8	29 ± 17†

PCW = pulmonary capillary wedge pressure.
*Values expressed as mean ± standard deviation (N = 22).
†Significantly higher than value at baseline and comparable to value at cardiac catherization.

TABLE 9-2. Jet and Left Atrial Dimensions Before and After Intraoperative Phenylephrine Administration*

Dimension	Baseline	Phenylephrine
Jet		
Length (cm)	2.3 ± 0.9	3.5 ± 1.2†
Width (cm)	1.2 ± 0.7	2.1 ± 0.7†
Circumference (cm)	6.3 ± 2.9	10.7 ± 3.3†
Area (cm^2)	2.3 ± 1.8	6.5 ± 3.5†
Left Atrium		
Length (cm)	6.1 ± 0.9	6.4 ± 0.7
Width (cm)	4.1 ± 0.6	4.2 ± 0.6
Circumference (cm)	18.4 ± 2.4	19.1 ± 1.8
Area (cm^2)	20.1 ± 5.1	22.1 ± 4.3†
Jet to left atrial ratio		
Length (%)	38 ± 15	55 ± 18†
Width (%)	28 ± 18	49 ± 16†
Circumference (%)	34 ± 15	56 ± 15†
Area (%)	11 ± 8	29 ± 13†

*Values expressed as mean ± standard deviation (N = 22).
†P < .05 compared with baseline value.

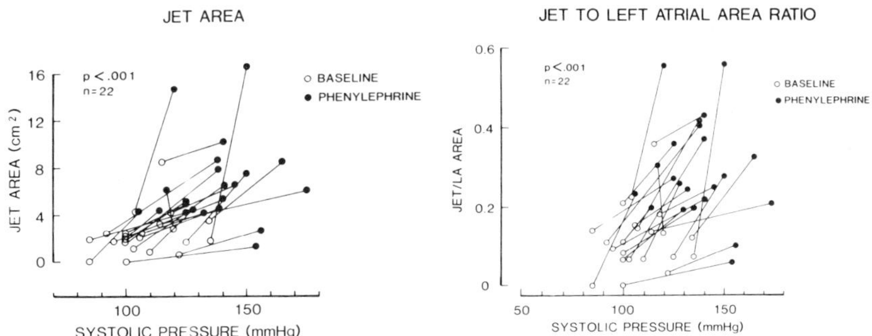

FIGURE 9-5. Impact of afterload on mitral regurgitant jet size. Increases in *systolic pressure* (horizontal axis) were associated with increases in *jet area* (left vertical axis) and *jet-to-left-atrial area* ratio (right vertical axis) (P<.001).

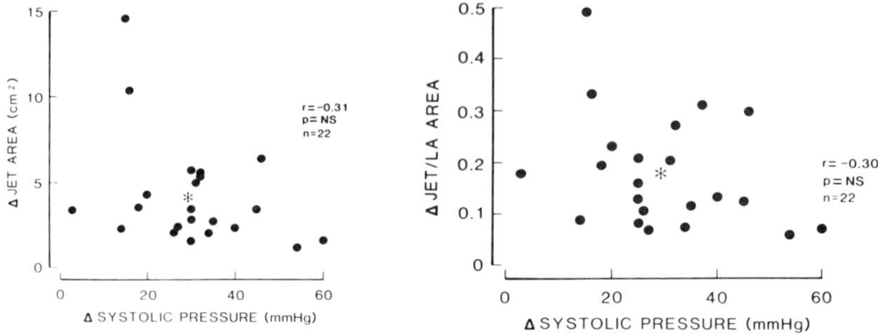

FIGURE 9-6. Poor correlation between magnitude of increase in *systolic pressure* (horizontal axis) and magnitude of increase in *jet area* (left verticle axis) or *jet-to-left-atrial area* ratio (right verticle axis). This finding implies that factors in addition to systolic pressure may influence jet size measurement by color Doppler.

geometry, including vortex flow and multiple jets, estimation of regurgitant volume from two-dimensional data, and temporal (dynamic) variation in jet size during systole. Systolic pressure is only one of many physiologic and technical factors that may influence jet size.

Accuracy of Regurgitation Grading

If appropriate attention is paid to adjustment of afterload and preload conditions to preoperative baseline or fixed reference levels, good agreement between angiographic and color Doppler evaluation of regurgitation is obtained (Figs. 9-7 and 9-8). Sensitivity is 94% and specificity 93% for detection of mitral regurgitation,[1] and the accuracy of tricuspid regurgitation grading is 88%.[2] Interobserver variability for grading of mitral or tricuspid regurgitation has been low, with both observers agreeing to within one grade in all patients.[2,5] Epicardial color Doppler thus provides a semiquantitative assessment of the severity of regurgitation comparable to that of angiography.

Comparison with Conventional Techniques

Previous studies have emphasized that atrial V waves are of limited value in assessing regurgitation severity.[6–8] During cardiac surgery, the V waves are subject to a wide variety of physiologic alterations due to

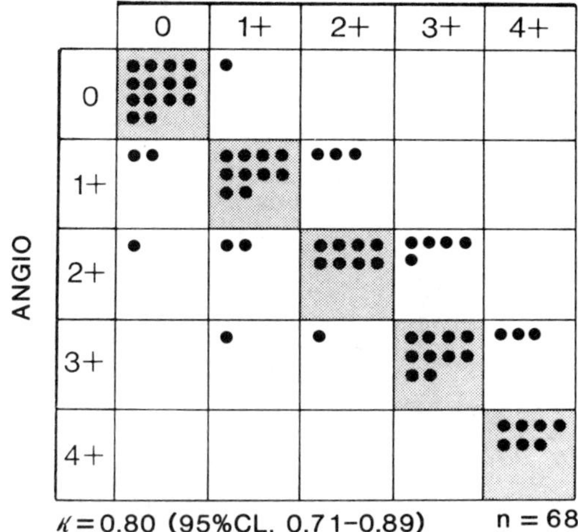

FIGURE 9-7. Agreement between color Doppler and left ventricular angiography for grading of mitral regurgitation. A kappa *(K)* value of 1.00 indicates perfect agreement, a value of zero indicates no or random agreement. A kappa value of 0.80 is considered very good agreement. *CL,* confidence limits.

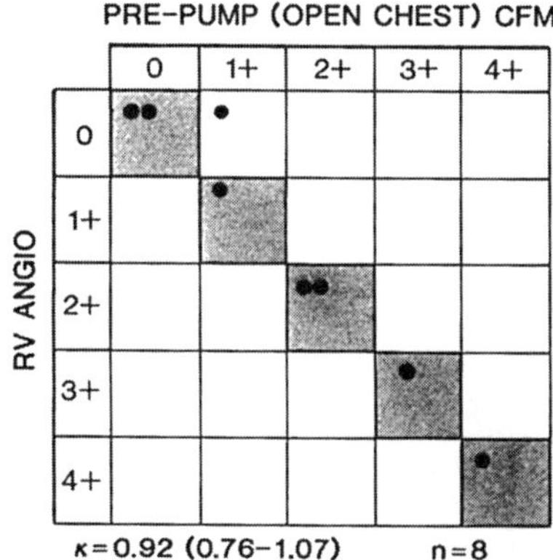

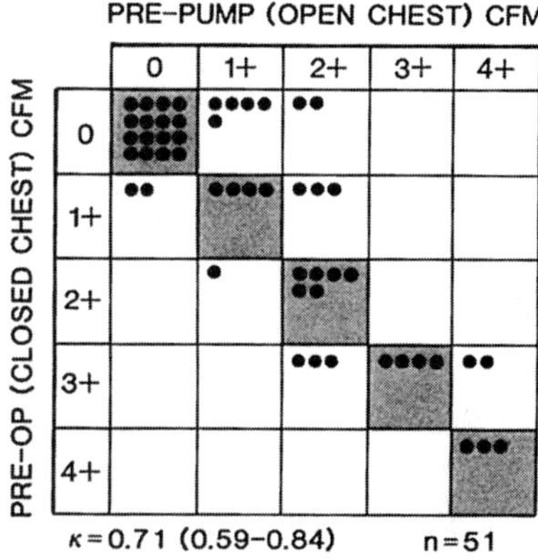

FIGURE 9-8. Agreement between color Doppler and angiography *(left)* and between preoperative and prepump color Doppler *(right)* for grading of tricuspid regurgitation. A kappa *(K)* value of 1.00 indicates perfect agreement, a value of zero indicates no or random agreement. A kappa value of 0.92 is considered excellent and 0.71 good agreement. Numbers in parentheses indicate confidence limits.

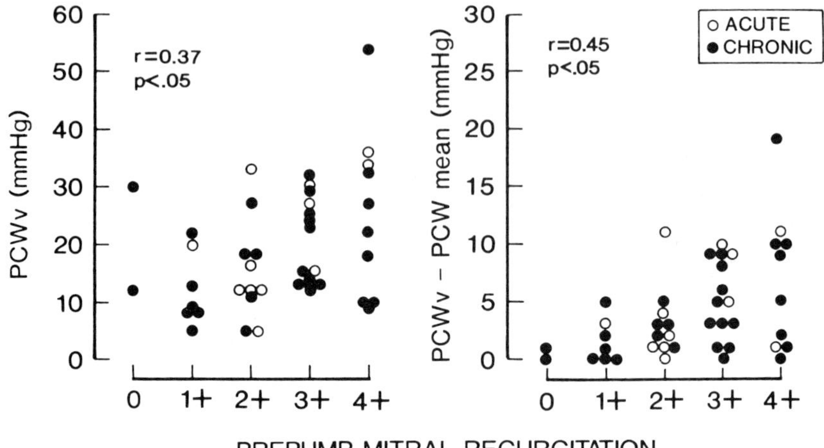

FIGURE 9-9. Poor correlation between color Doppler grade of mitral regurgitation and pulmonary capillary wedge *(PCW)* V wave when measured as either the absolute magnitude *(left)* or its height above the mean *(right).* Although statistically significant, the correlation coefficients were low. Stratification into acute and chronic mitral regurgitation did not consistently improve the correlations.

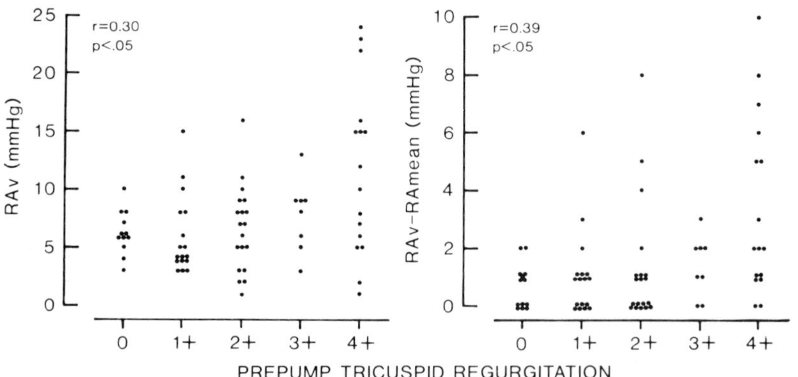

FIGURE 9-10. Poor correlation between color Doppler grade of tricuspid regurgitation and right atrial *(RA)* V wave when measured either as the absolute magnitude *(left)* or its height above the mean *(right).* Although statistically significant, the correlation coefficients were low.

TABLE 9-3. Fluid Filling of the Arrested Ventricle*

Valve Tested	Fluid Leakage	Color Doppler Regurgitation Grade				
		0	*1+*	*2+*	*3+*	*4+*
Mitral	none (n = 10)†	4	3	2	1	0
	mild (n = 5)‡	2	1	1	1	0
Tricuspid	none (n = 4)§	1	1	2	0	0
	mild (n = 8)‖	2	3	1	1	1
	moderate (n = 1)‖	0	0	1	0	0

*A poor correlation was seen between fluid leakage and color Doppler grade of regurgitation for both the mitral and tricuspid valves.
†False negative rate (no leak, with 2+ to 4+ regurgitation) 30% (3/10).
‡False positive rate (leak, with no regurgitation) 40% (2/5).
§False negative rate 50% (2/4).
‖False positive rate 22% (2/9).

the effects of anesthesia, ischemia, pericardiotomy, use of pressors or vasodilators, and shifts in interstitial sodium and water; these factors may change atrial size and compliance, as well as influence preload and afterload conditions,[9–13] potentially invalidating the V wave as a useful indicator of regurgitation severity. In fact, it was found that the atrial V wave correlated poorly with the color Doppler grade of regurgitation, both before (Figs. 9-9 and 9-10) and after cardiopulmonary bypass.[1,2]

Fluid filling of the arrested ventricle by means of a bulb syringe is a commonly employed method of assessing mitral or tricuspid regurgitation during cardiac surgery. The use of a bulb syringe, although simple, produces a highly variable pressure source and may induce artifactual regurgitation by distortion of the valve or use of excessive force; in addition, the grading of regurgitation is highly subjective. Because valve closure requires a dynamic and complex interaction among the valve leaflets, chordae tendineae, papillary muscles, and adjacent myocardium, competence may not be adequately assessed in the arrested heart. It has been found that fluid filling of the arrested ventricle as a means of testing valve competency correlates poorly with regurgitation grade by color Doppler (Table 9-3).

EVALUATION OF THE VALVE REPAIR PATIENT

In patients with mitral or tricuspid regurgitation, echocardiography combined with Doppler color-flow mapping provides information with immediate relevance to the need for valve repair, the feasibility of repair, and the planning of the surgical procedure. Often, the etiologic basis of the valve disease (myxomatous degeneration, infective endocarditis, and rheumatic, ischemic, or congenital causes) can be determined, and, together with the severity of the regurgitation, this information facilitates decision-making regarding the need for surgical inspection of the valve and adjacent structures. In patients with aortic valve disease, a special issue relates to sizing of the aortic annulus if homograft replacement is anticipated. Following valve repair, echocardiography combined with color Doppler is especially useful for evaluating the presence and severity of residual regurgitation and for identifying complications associated with the repair procedure.

Annulus

Dilation of the annulus results from chronic mitral or tricuspid regurgitation and often occurs in association with atrial enlargement. In addition, the annulus loses its elliptical shape, becoming more circular. Annular dilation in turn makes the valve leaflets coapt poorly and eventually produces valvular incompetence. Reestablishment of a normal annular size and shape can reduce or eliminate valvular regurgitation. The need for an annulus-reducing procedure, therefore, can be determined by echocardiographic assessment of the annular dimensions (Fig. 9-11).[4]

In patients who have had ring annuloplasty, the ring can be imaged echocardiographically in long- and short-axis views (Figs. 9-12 and 9-13). The cross-sectional area available for flow can be determined directly from the short-axis view by planimetry of the internal orifice of the ring. Additionally, pulsed- or continuous-wave Doppler velocity measurements can be used to determine the pressure half-time of transvalvular diastolic flow; the valve area can be calculated from the formula A = 220/pressure half-time (in milliseconds). In general, the orifice area should be greater than 1.0 cm^2 per square meter of body surface area. Overcorrection of regurgitation by insertion of too small a ring can produce functional stenosis.

Left ventricular outflow tract obstruction is a well-described complication that occurs in 4.5% to 6.0% of patients who undergo mitral annuloplasty with a rigid Carpentier-Edwards ring.[14,15] This finding is associated with systolic anterior motion of the mitral leaflets; no patient has had septal hypertrophy. Left ventricular outflow tract obstruction has not been described after suture annuloplasty or annuloplasty using the flexible Duran ring.

In patients who are candidates for homograft replacement of the aortic valve, echocardiography can be used to determine the size of the

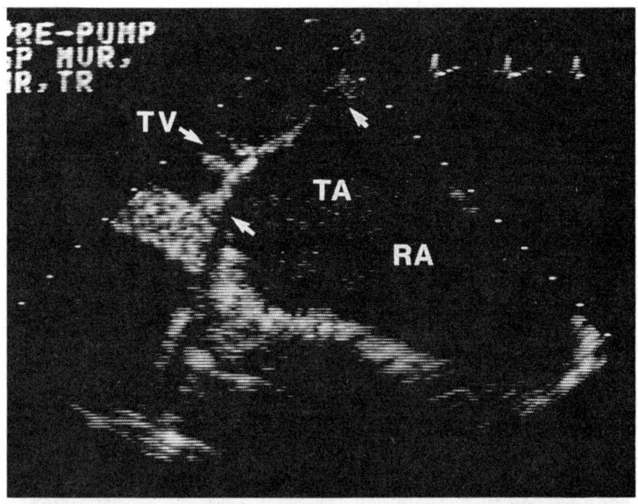

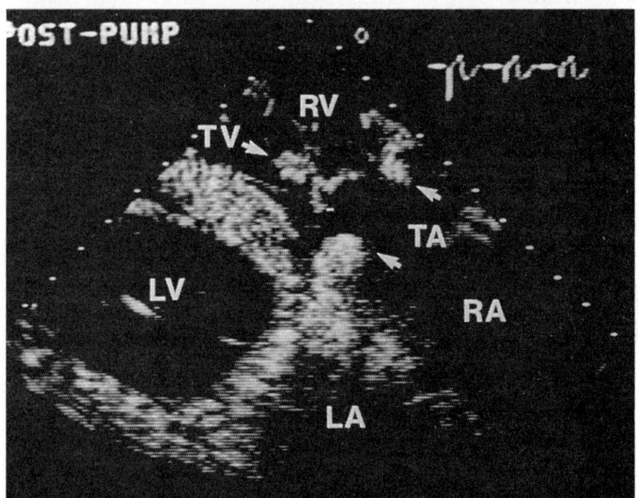

FIGURE 9-11. Dilated tricuspid annulus and right atrium before repair *(upper photo).* After tricuspid annuloplasty with a Carpentier-Edwards ring, the tricuspid annulus is markedly reduced *(lower photo).* Epicardial long-axis equivalent view of right ventricle *(RV),* tricuspid valve *(TV),* annulus *(TA),* and right atrium *(RA). LA,* left atrium; *LV,* left ventricle.

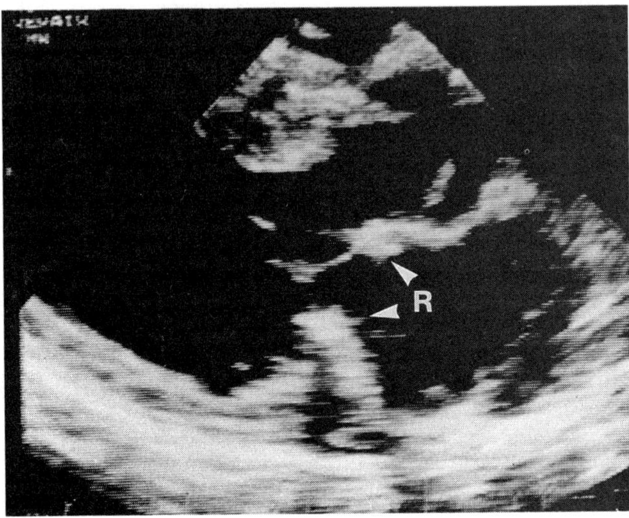

FIGURE 9-12. Mitral annuloplasty with a Carpentier-Edwards prosthetic ring. The annuloplasty ring *(R)* is seen in cross-section at the base of the anterior and posterior leaflets. Epicardial parasternal-equivalent long-axis view during systole.

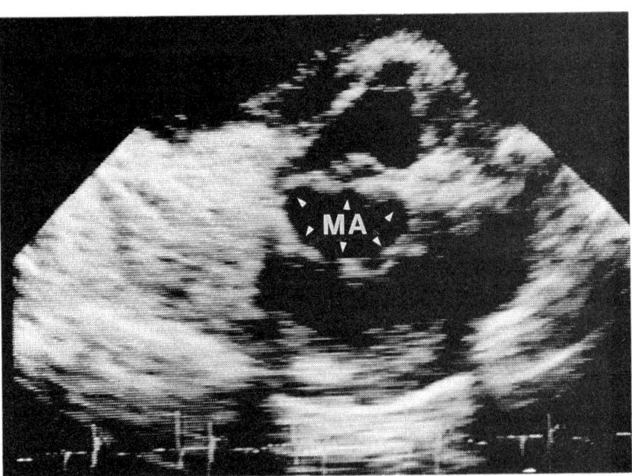

FIGURE 9-13. Mitral annuloplasty *(MA)* with a Carpentier-Edwards prosthetic ring, imaged in an epicardial parasternal-equivalent short-axis view. The elliptical shape of the annuloplasty ring *(arrows)* is apparent.

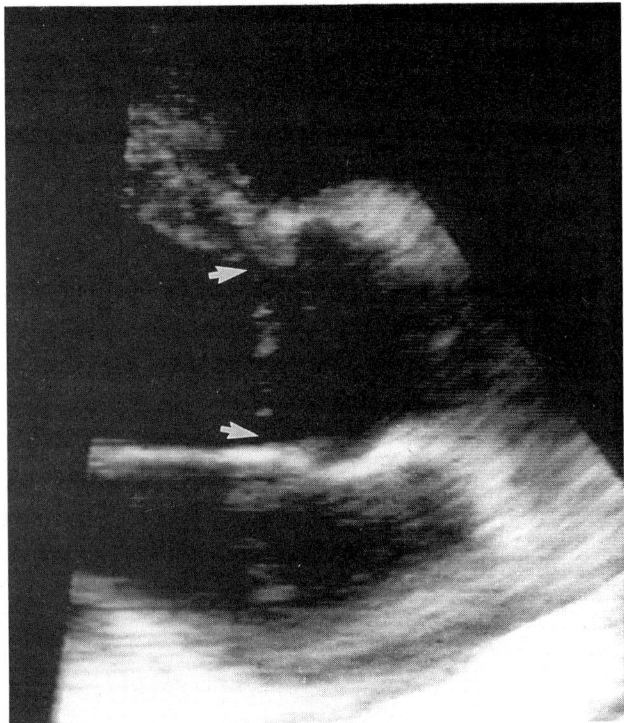

FIGURE 9-14. Measurement of aortic annulus diameter. The aortic annulus *(arrows)* is located at the base of the aortic leaflets, just above the left ventricular outflow tract. Epicardial parasternal-equivalent long-axis view.

aortic annulus. The annulus is measured at the base of the aortic leaflets, at the end of the left ventricular outflow tract (Fig. 9-14). This measurement helps determine whether appropriately sized homografts are available for the patient. After homograft replacement of the aortic valve, either residual regurgitation or stenosis may occur, and these complications can be identified readily by epicardial color Doppler echocardiography.

Leaflets

In patients with mitral or tricuspid regurgitation, myxomatous degeneration may produce ballooning and scalloping of the valve leaflets or localized area of thinning or thickening, all of which can be identified echocardiographically. Marked prolapse or leaflet malalignment may be present, resulting from chordal elongation. In patients with active endocarditis, vegetations may be attached to the leaflets or chords. Ruptured major chordae may be seen in the atrium during systole. With rheumatic valve disease, thickening or calcification of the leaflets, restriction of leaflet motion, and a variable degree of shortening and thickening of the subvalvular apparatus may be identified. In patients with regurgitation due to coronary artery disease, the leaflets and chords appear normal (Color plate 7).

Thus, the pathologic changes in the leaflets or chords and the etiologic basis of the regurgitation can often be identified echocardiographically. This information helps to plan the surgical procedure. For example, the finding of a torn chord or prolapsed leaflet in a patient with mitral regurgitation and coronary artery disease may entail a more complicated mitral valve procedure than was initially anticipated.

After repair, residual regurgitation should be evaluated with hemodynamic conditions similar to the prepump study. In patients with mitral regurgitation, phenylephrine should be administered if the systolic pressure is more than 15 mm Hg below a prior baseline or fixed reference level, to increase the systolic pressure to an appropriate level. Fluids should be administered as needed to adjust preload conditions.

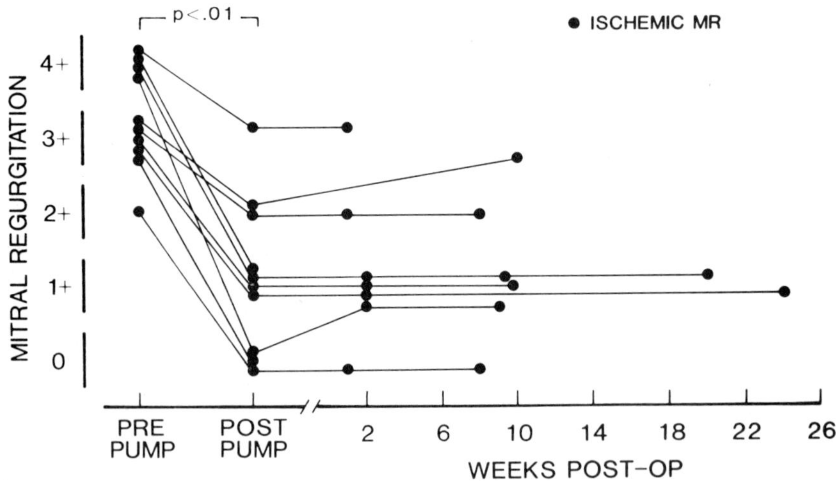

FIGURE 9-15. Longitudinal study of mitral regurgitation *(MR)* after mitral valve repair. No significant change in the average grade of regurgitation was found after the initial postpump study. The vertical axis depicts the color Doppler grade of regurgitation, and the horizontal axis is the time at which the study was performed.

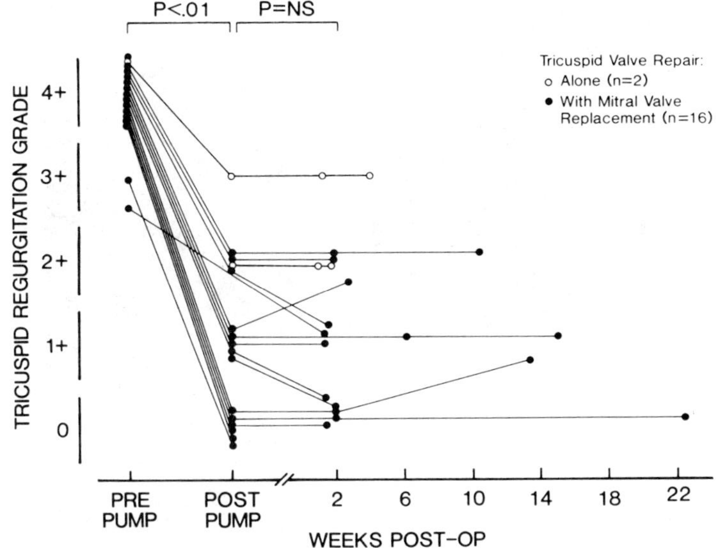

FIGURE 9-16. Longitudinal study of tricuspid regurgitation after tricuspid valve repair. There was no significant change in the average grade of regurgitation was found after the initial postpump study. The vertical axis depicts the color Doppler grade of regurgitation, and the horizontal axis is the time at which the study was performed. *(Czer LSC, Maurer G, Bolger A et al: Tricuspid valve repair: Operative and follow up evaluation by Doppler color flow mapping. J Thorac Cardiovasc Surg 98:101, 1989)*

The cause of residual regurgitation often can be identified by careful echocardiographic evaluation of the leaflets and chords. For example, continued prolapse despite ring annuloplasty may indicate insufficient chordal shortening. Residual regurgitation after repair of a cleft mitral leaflet may indicate inadequate closure of the cleft (Color plate 8). Follow-up studies after mitral or tricuspid valve repair have demonstrated no significant change in the grade of regurgitation from the postpump to subsequent postoperative evaluations (Figs. 9-15 and 9-16), unless there has been an intervening event. Thus, the immediate postpump study is a good predictor of the long-term results of valve repair.

Papillary Muscles and Wall Motion

Segmental thinning of the myocardium, atresia of the papillary muscles, and dyskinetic wall segments are indicative of prior infarction. Segmental wall motion abnormalities (other than dyskinesia) may be

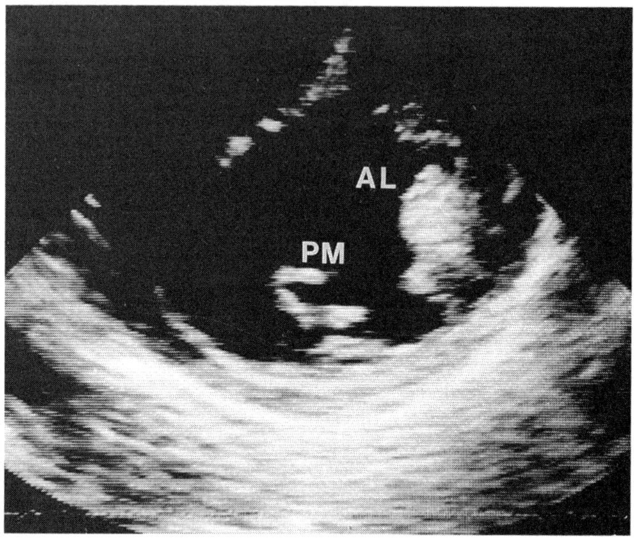

FIGURE 9-17. Posteromedial papillary muscle atresia associated with inferior infarction and thinning of the inferior wall. Epicardial parasternal-equivalent short-axis view of left ventricle at papillary muscle level. *PM,* posteromedial papillary muscle; *AL,* anterolateral papillary muscle.

produced by reversible ischemia or infarction. These findings may be helpful in patients with mitral regurgitation to establish coronary artery disease as the cause of the regurgitation. Atretic papillary muscles can be identified by their diminutive size and increased echocardiographic density on short-axis imaging (Fig. 9-17).

Direction of Regurgitant Jet

Jet direction provides corroborative evidence of leaflet prolapse and chordal elongation. For example, in a patient with mitral regurgitation, a jet directed under the anterior mitral leaflet is associated with prolapse of the posterior leaflet. Similarly, a jet directed along the inferior or free posterolateral wall of the left atrium is associated with anterior leaflet prolapse.

Origin of Regurgitant Jet

In patients with mitral regurgitation due to coronary artery disease, the origin of the jet in relation to the commissure may help guide surgical decision making. The mitral commissure may be divided arbitrarily into thirds: the inferior portion (adjacent to the inferior wall of the left ventricle), the middle portion, and the superior portion (adjacent to the anterolateral wall of the left ventricle). The mitral commissure and the origin of the jet can be imaged from the epicardial parasternal-equivalent short-axis view. It has been found that ischemic mitral regurgitation originates from the inferior commissure (42%) or from the central portion of the commissure (52%) in most patients.[16] An example of a jet that originates from the inferior portion of the mitral commissure is shown in Figure 9-18.

The origin of the jet correlates with the success of valve repair by suture annuloplasty. Jets that originated from the inferior commissure

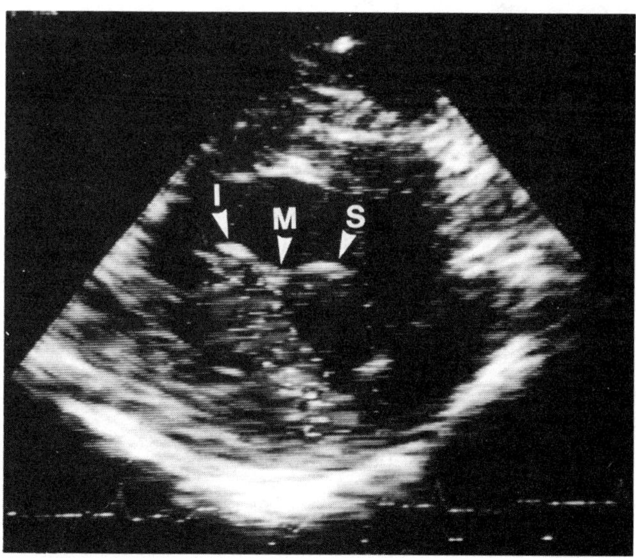

FIGURE 9-18. Regurgitant jet originating from inferior commissure of mitral valve. Commissural location marked as inferior *(I)*, middle *(M)*, and superior *(S)*. Epicardial parasternal-equivalent short-axis view at base of mitral leaflets.

that were treated by a Kay-Zubiate suture annuloplasty had a 90% success rate, whereas central jets treated by the same technique had only a 67% success rate.[16] The latter patients may have an improved success rate with ring annuloplasty.

ASSESSMENT OF VENTRICULAR SEPTAL DEFECTS AFTER ACUTE MYOCARDIAL INFARCTION

Rupture of the interventricular septum may occur after inferior or anterior myocardial infarction, creating a muscular septal defect with left-to-right shunting of blood flow between the ventricles. With inferior infarctions, the defect is often in the low septum, adjacent to the inferior wall of the left ventricle (Fig. 9-19). After anterior infarction, the defect is usually in the apical portion of the septum (Fig. 9-20). Multiple defects may occur. Intraoperative echocardiography is useful for identifying the precise location and number of defects; in addition, intramyocardial hemorrhage and edema may be identified by fracturing of the tissue and changes in the echocardiographic tissue density, respectively (see Fig. 9-19). Doppler color-flow mapping can identify multiple shunts when all of the defects are not obvious echocardiographically.

Immediately after repair, Doppler color-flow mapping may identify small jets of high velocity flow, which represent leakage through suture holes in the patch. On later follow-up studies, the small jets have not been seen; the conclusion, therefore, is that these small suture leaks are eventually sealed by clot formation or endothelialization. Larger leaks and flow between two patches of a sandwich-type septal defect repair are definitely abnormal and may indicate the need for revision of the repair.[17,18]

EVALUATION OF CORONARY ARTERIES AND BYPASS GRAFTS

Epicardial imaging of coronary arteries and coronary bypass grafts requires high-frequency transducers to provide adequate spatial resolution for good anatomic definition. A 12 MHz linear scanning transducer (Surgiscan, Biosound Corporation, Indianapolis, Indiana) is available for two-dimensional ultrasound imaging. This device has been useful for detection of technical errors and inadequacies in bypass graft anastomoses and in the evaluation of the native coronary arteries at the sites of anastomoses.[19]

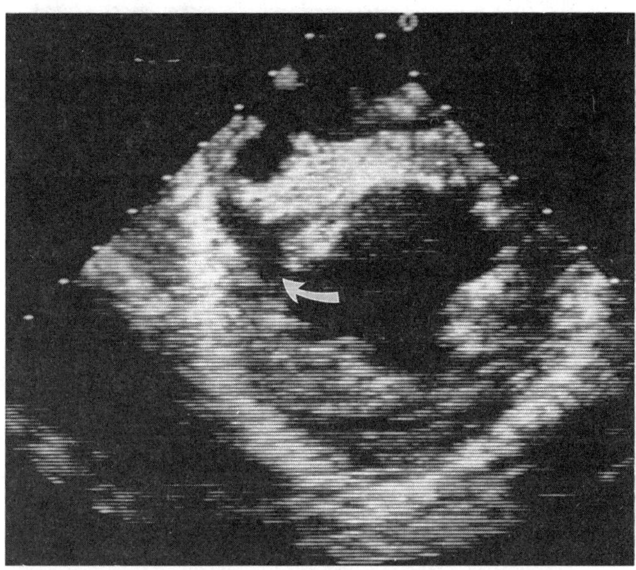

FIGURE 9-19. Ventricular septal defect after inferior myocardial infarction. A channel between the interventricular septum and the diaphragmatic wall of the left ventricle is present and represents an acutely ruptured ventricular septum that occurred as a complication of an inferior myocardial infarction *(arrow)*. The edge of the defect is irregular due to intramyocardial hemorrhage and dissection of the ventricular septum. Epicardial parasternal-equivalent short-axis view of the left ventricle at papillary muscle level.

Epicardial echocardiography has been found useful in patients who are undergoing excimer laser angioplasty of the coronary arteries during cardiac surgery (Fig. 9-21). In these patients, epicardial ultrasound has provided precise localization of high-grade stenosis, has aided guidewire and excimer laser catheter placement, and has enabled immediate evaluation of the residual lesion after laser angioplasty.[20] Potential complications of the procedure, such as dissection or gas formation, can be detected intraoperatively. Tissue characterization of the arterial wall may help distinguish different types of atherosclerotic plaque.

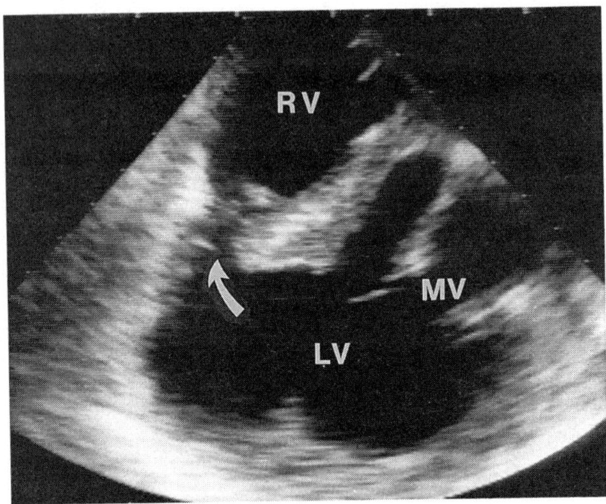

FIGURE 9-20. Ventricular septal defect after anterior myocardial infarction. A channel *(arrow)* appears between the distal interventricular septum and the apex of the left ventricle, representing an acutely ruptured ventricular septum as a consequence of anterior infarction. An apical aneurysm *(lower left of image)* is evident from a prior infarction. Epicardial image obtained from anterior surface of right ventricle *(RV)*, with transducer angled toward apex of left ventricle *(LV)*. *MV*, mitral valve.

A 7.5 MHz prototype transducer under development allows color Doppler imaging of blood flow within the artery or bypass graft (Fig. 9-22). Quantitation of blood flow within the coronary artery or bypass graft may be possible with this instrument.

CONCLUSION

Epicardial echocardiography with Doppler color-flow mapping provides valuable anatomic and physiologic information that aids intraoperative decision making. In the patient with suspected regurgitation, this technique can be used to determine the severity of regurgitation, the impact of physiologic interventions on regurgitation severity, the

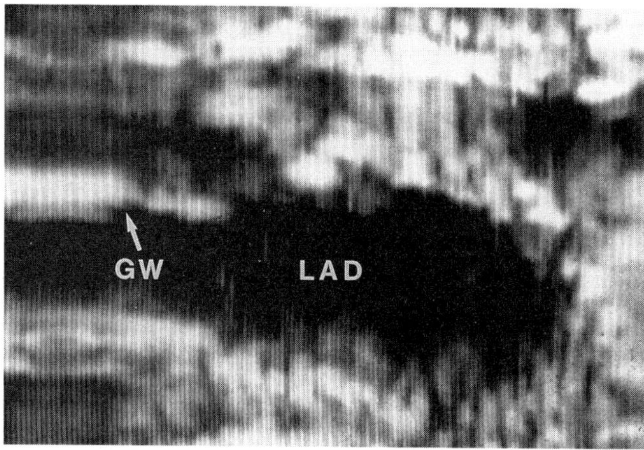

FIGURE 9-21. Epicardial echocardiographic image of left anterior descending *(LAD)* coronary artery. A guidewire *(GW)* is seen within the lumen of the artery, over which a laser catheter was passed for ablation of a subtotal coronary stenosis. Epicardial imaging ensured proper placement of the guidewire and laser catheter. A 12 MHz transducer was used.

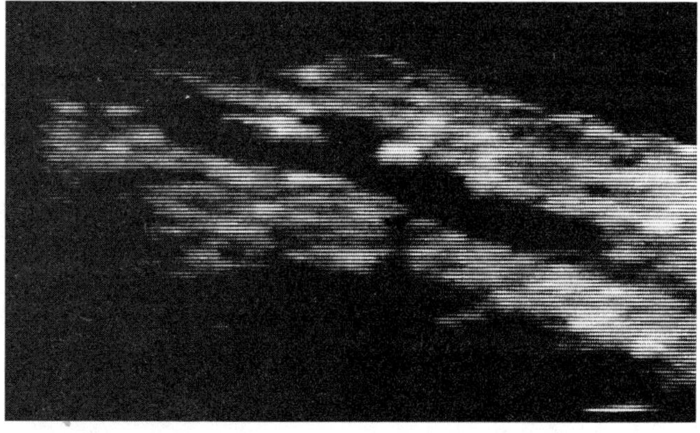

FIGURE 9-22. Epicardial image of atherosclerotic right coronary artery. Multiple projections into the lumen represent atherosclerotic plaque. A prototype 7.5 MHz transducer was used.

presence of associated lesions, and the state of ventricular function. In the valve repair candidate, this technique can be used to answer important clinical questions about, for example, the morphologic basis of the regurgitant lesion, the feasibility of repair, the adequacy of the surgical procedure after repair, and the presence of any associated complications such as outflow tract obstruction. This technique is also helpful in the evaluation of patients with a suspected ventricular septal defect after myocardial infarction, particularly for localization of the site of the defect, detection of multiple shunts, and evaluation of residual shunting after repair. In patients with coronary atherosclerosis, epicardial echocardiography is useful for characterization of stenosis and atheromas, for guidance and evaluation of interventional intracoronary procedures during cardiac surgery, and for assessment of the integrity of bypass graft anastomoses.

References

1. Czer LSC, Maurer G, Bolger AF et al: Intraoperative evaluation of mitral regurgitation by Doppler color flow mapping. Circulation 76 (suppl):108, 1987
2. Czer LSC, Maurer G, Bolger A et al: Tricuspid valve repair: Operative and follow-up evaluation by Doppler color flow mapping. J Thorac Cardiovasc Surg 98:101, 1989
3. Helmcke F, Nanda NC, Hsiung MC et al: Color Doppler assessment of mitral regurgitation with orthogonal planes. Circulation 75:175, 1987
4. Chopra HK, Nanda NC, Fan P et al: Can two-dimensional echocardiography and Doppler color flow mapping identify the need for tricuspid valve repair? J Am Coll Cardiol 14:1266, 1989
5. Maurer G, Czer LSC, Chaux A et al: Intraoperative Doppler color flow mapping for assessment of valve repair for mitral regurgitation. Am J Cardiol 60:333, 1987
6. Fuchs RM, Heuser RR, Yin FCP, Brinker JA: Limitations of pulmonary wedge V waves in diagnosing mitral regurgitation. Am J Cardiol 49:849, 1982
7. Braunwald E, Awe WC: The syndrome of severe mitral regurgitation with normal left atrial pressure. Circulation 27:29, 1963
8. Cohen SR, Sell JE, McIntosh CL, Clark RE: Tricuspid regurgitation in patients with acquired, chronic, pure mitral regurgitation. Part I. Prevalence, diagnosis, and comparison of preoperative clinical and hemodynamic features in patients with and without tricuspid regurgitation. J Thorac Cardiovasc Surg 94:481, 1987
9. Mammana RB, Hiro S, Levitsky S, Thomas PS, Plachetka J: Inaccuracy of pulmonary capillary wedge pressure when compared to left atrial pressure in the early postsurgical period. J Thorac Cardiovasc Surg 84:420, 1982
10. Ellis RJ, Mangano DT, Van Dyke DC: Relationship of wedge pressure to

end-diastolic volume in patients undergoing myocardial revascularization. J Thorac Cardiovasc Surg 78:605, 1979
11. Lappas D, Lell WA, Gabel JC, Civetta JM, Lowenstein E: Indirect measurement of left-atrial pressure in surgical patients: Pulmonary-capillary wedge and pulmonary artery diastolic pressures compared with left-atrial pressure. Anesthesiology 38:394, 1973
12. Cohen ST, Sell JE, McIntosh CL, Clark RE: Tricuspid regurgitation in patients with acquired, chronic, pure mitral regurgitation. Part II. Nonoperative management, tricuspid valve annuloplasty, and tricuspid valve replacement. J Thorac Cardiovasc Surg 94:488, 1987
13. Goldman ME, Guarino T, Fuster V, Mindich B: The necessity for tricuspid valve repair can be determined intraoperatively by two-dimensional echocardiography. J Thorac Cardiovasc Surg 94:542, 1987
14. Mihaileanu S, Marino JP, Chauvaud S et al: Left ventricular outflow obstruction after mitral valve repair (Carpentier's technique): Proposed mechanisms of disease. Circulation 78 (suppl):78, 1988
15. Schiavone WA, Cosgrove DM, Lever HM, Stewart WJ, Salcedo EE: Long-term follow-up of patients with left ventricular outflow tract obstruction after Carpentier ring mitral valvuloplasty. Circulation 78 (suppl):60, 1988
16. Czer LSC, Maurer G, Bolger A et al: Ischemic mitral regurgitation: Comparative evaluation of revascularization versus repair by Doppler color flow mapping. Circulation 76 (suppl):389, 1987
17. Maurer G, Czer LSC: Intraoperative Doppler color flow mapping. In Nanda NC (ed): Textbook of Color Doppler Echocardiography, pp. 258–270. Philadelphia, Lea & Febiger, 1989
18. Maurer G, Czer LSC, Shah PK, Chaux A: Assessment by Doppler color flow mapping of ventricular septal defect after acute myocardial infarction. Am J Cardiol 64:668, 1989
19. Hiratzka LF, McPherson DD, Lamberth WC et al: Intraoperative evaluation of coronary artery bypass graft anastomoses with high-frequency epicardial echocardiography: Experimental validation and initial patient studies. Circulation 73:1199, 1986
20. Wong WS, Czer LSC, Blanche C, Grundfest WS, Maurer G: Epicardial coronary echo guidance of intraoperative laser angioplasty. Circulation 80 (suppl):564, 1989

Martin D. Abel
Rick A. Nishimura

10 The Intraoperative Use of Pulsed-Wave Doppler Echocardiography

THE DOPPLER EFFECT

When a train is moving toward the station, the pitch of its whistle increases because the wavelength of sound is compressed relative to one's ear (Fig. 10-1). When the train moves beyond the station, the wavelength of sound is increased relative to one's ear, and the frequency or pitch decreases correspondingly. The change in the frequency of sound that occurs because of relative movement between source and observer is termed the Doppler shift or Doppler frequency and was first described by Christian Johann Doppler (1803–1853), an Austrian physicist.[1] The Doppler shift can be expressed by Equation 10-1,

$$\Delta f = f_r - f_t \qquad (10\text{-}1)$$

where Δf equals the Doppler frequency shift; f_r the frequency received or the reflected frequency; and f_t the frequency of transmitted sound. The Doppler phenomenon is common to all types of waves in which the source and the receiver are moving relative to each other.[2]

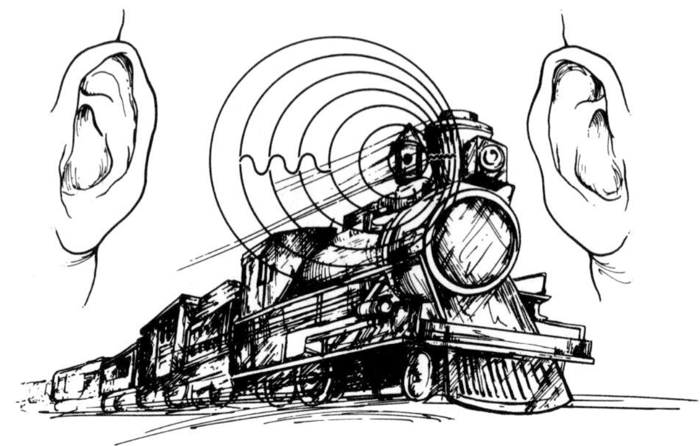

FIGURE 10-1. **Schematic diagram of the Doppler effect. As a train, which is the source of the emitting sound wave, moves toward the receiving ear, there is a decrease in the wavelength of sound and an increase in the pitch of its whistle. Conversely, when the train moves away from the receiving ear, the wavelength of sound is increased and the frequency of the pitch decreases.** *(Nishimura RA, Callahan MJ, Warnes CA: Echocardiography. In Giuliani ER, Fuster V, Gersh BJ, McGoon DC, McGoon MD (eds): Cardiology: Fundamentals and Practice, 2nd ed. Chicago, Year Book Medical Publishers [in press], by permission of Mayo Foundation)*

ULTRASOUND

Ultrasound employs sound waves with a frequency well above the audible level, usually in the range of 1 to 10 MHz. In the clinical application of ultrasound technology, backscattered sound is used to generate two-dimensional images, while the Doppler shift is used to measure the velocity of blood flow. The Doppler effect is used in clinical medicine to measure the velocity of blood within the cardiovascular system. In this situation, the moving red blood cells reflect the sound emitted by a transmitter. The difference in frequency between the sound emitted by the transducer and that received by the receiver is a function of the red blood cell velocity and is accurately measured by ultrasound equipment, which records it as a Doppler frequency shift.

BLOOD-FLOW VELOCITY

Blood-flow velocity can be determined from the Doppler Equation 10-2,

$$\Delta f = 2 f_t \frac{V\cos\theta}{c} \tag{10-2}$$

where Δf equals Doppler frequency shift, which is measured by the ultrasonograph; f_t is the transmitted frequency and is specific to a given transducer; V is the velocity of red blood cells; θ is the angle between the vector of blood-flow velocity and the incident angle of the ultrasound beam; and c is the speed of sound in biological tissue ($1{,}560\ \mathrm{m \cdot s^{-1}}$).[1]

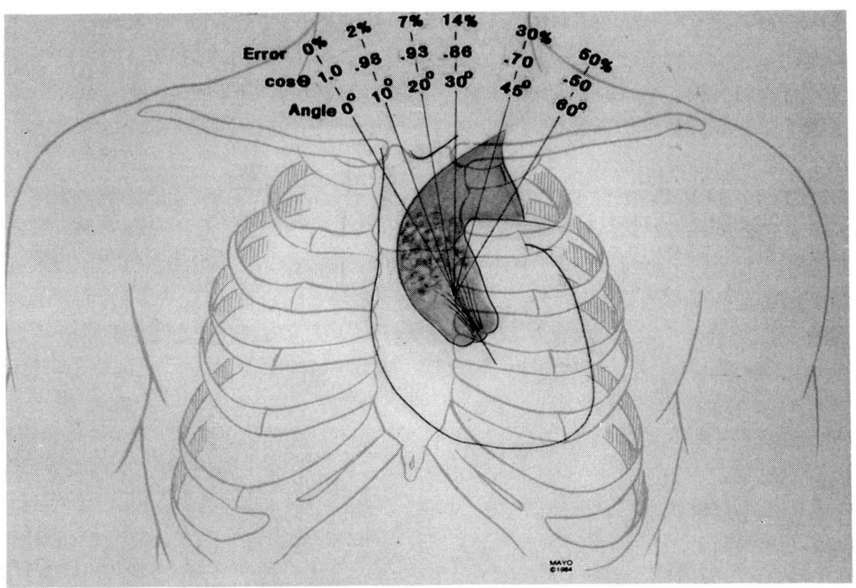

FIGURE 10-2. Schematic diagram demonstrates the effect of the angle of incidence on the Doppler equation. The cosine of θ and the angle of incidence between the Doppler beam and the blood velocity jet are shown, with the resultant underestimation of the true velocity *(error).* As the angle θ is greater, the angle of incidence and underestimation of the blood-flow velocity is greater. *(Nishimura RA, Miller FA, Callahan MJ et al: Doppler echocardiography: Theory, instrumentation, technique and application. Mayo Clin Proc 60:321, 1985)*

As the angle θ approaches 0 degrees, cos θ approaches unity. Thus, if the angle θ is minimized by reducing the incident angle between the vector of blood velocity and the ultrasound beam, then the radial velocity ($V\cos\theta$) will be equal to the velocity of blood measured by the ultrasound equipment (V). If the angle θ is less than 20 degrees, the error introduced by it is relatively small. However, if the angle of incidence is large, this error becomes significant. To illustrate this effect, consider the following example using Figures 10-2 and 10-3, and Table 10-1. If the true velocity of blood-flow is 4 $m \cdot s^{-1}$ and the angle between the ultrasound beam and the vector of blood-flow velocity is 50 degrees, then the measured velocity of the blood-flow will be 2.6 $m \cdot s^{-1}$, a 35% underestimation. If the angle θ were only 20 degrees, then the measured velocity would be 3.8 $m \cdot s^{-1}$ (only a 5% underestimation) and would provide clinically useful information. It is imperative that the ultrasound beam be as parallel as possible to the direction of the blood-flow velocity vector to ensure that its maximum velocity is determined.

ULTRASOUND DOPPLER MODES AND INSTRUMENTATION

Commercially available ultrasonographic equipment is capable of using continuous-wave or pulsed-wave Doppler modalities with or without simultaneous two-dimensional imaging. An audible signal of the Dopp-

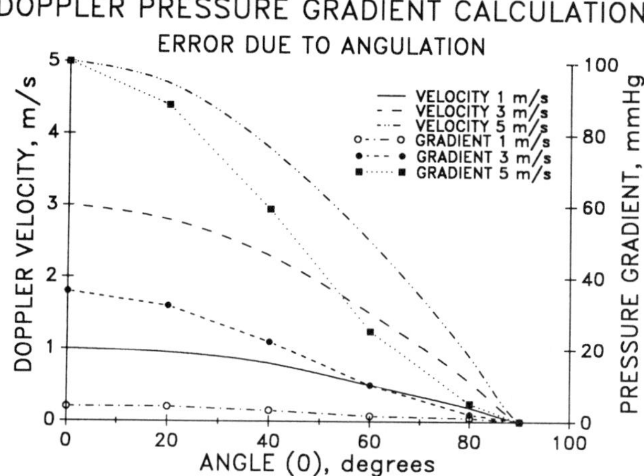

FIGURE 10-3. Diagram illustrates the interrelationship of Doppler velocity, angle of incidence, and pressure gradient.

TABLE 10-1. **Error Due to Angle of Doppler Beam to Velocity Jet**

VELOCITY								
Angle θ	cos θ	1 m/s	2 m/s	3 m/s	4 m/s	5 m/s	6 m/s	Error (%)*
0	1.00	1.00	2.00	3.00	4.00	5.00	6.00	0
10	0.98	0.98	1.97	2.95	3.94	4.92	5.91	2
20	0.94	0.94	1.88	2.82	3.76	4.70	5.64	6
30	0.87	0.87	1.73	2.60	3.46	4.33	5.20	13
40	0.77	0.77	1.53	2.30	3.06	3.83	4.60	23
50	0.64	0.64	1.29	1.93	2.57	3.21	3.86	36
60	0.50	0.50	1.00	1.50	2.00	2.50	3.00	50
70	0.34	0.34	0.68	1.03	1.37	1.71	2.05	66
80	0.17	0.17	0.35	0.52	0.69	0.87	1.04	83
90	0.00	0.00	0.00	0.00	0.00	0.00	0.00	100
PRESSURE GRADIENT (mm Hg)								
Angle θ	cos θ	1 m/s	2 m/s	3 m/s	4 m/s	5 m/s	6 m/s	Error (%)*
0	1.00	4.00	16.00	36.00	64.00	100.00	144.00	0
10	0.98	3.88	15.52	34.91	62.07	96.98	139.66	3
20	0.94	3.53	14.13	31.79	56.51	88.30	127.16	12
30	0.87	3.00	12.00	27.00	48.00	75.00	108.00	25
40	0.77	2.35	9.39	21.13	37.56	58.68	84.50	41
50	0.64	1.65	6.61	14.87	26.44	41.32	59.50	59
60	0.50	1.00	4.00	9.00	16.00	25.00	36.00	75
70	0.34	0.47	1.87	4.21	7.49	11.70	16.84	88
80	0.17	0.12	0.48	1.09	1.93	3.02	4.34	97
90	0.00	0.00	0.00	0.00	0.00	0.00	0.00	100

*Error is the percentage error between the measured velocity or pressure gradient and the tone value.

ler frequency shift is used to discriminate turbulent and laminar flow and facilitates positioning of the transducer. Data that usually are displayed include the electrocardiogram, which may be used to time the Doppler velocity signal, and a spectral display of blood velocity, in which the velocity is displayed on the y axis and time on the x axis.[3] By convention, flow away from the transducer is displayed below the baseline and flow toward the transducer is displayed above the baseline. If the envelope of the velocity spectrum has a sharp, well-defined border with minimal shading underneath, laminar flow is present. Shading underneath the envelope indicates that a wide range of velocities are present in the jet, often associated with turbulent flow.

Pulsed-Wave Mode

A single ultrasound crystal serves as both the emitter of the ultrasound and as the receiver of the reflected ultrasound. Short bursts or pulses of ultrasound are emitted with a particular frequency, the pulse-repetition frequency, and reception of the backscattered sound occurs between these pulses. Because transmission time is a function of the distance between the transducer and the blood-flow velocity jet, pulsed-wave Doppler can be time gated so that only the velocities at a particular depth are analyzed. This ability allows depth or range localization of the blood-flow velocity jet. Frequently a pulsed-wave Doppler examination is combined with a simultaneous two-dimensional echocardiographic examination to position a sample volume (the depth locator) precisely within a cardiac chamber, for example, at the level of the aortic valve (Fig. 10-4).

The maximum frequency shift that can be quantitated accurately by pulsed-wave Doppler techniques without depth ambiguity is equal to half the pulse-repetition frequency, a frequency shift that is termed the Nyquist frequency or limit.[4] This limit is necessary because the backscattered signal must be received before the next pulse is emitted. As the depth of the sample volume increases, the pulse-repetition frequency must be reduced to allow enough time for signal reception, and the result is a further decrease in the maximum Doppler frequency shift that can be recorded. If the frequency shift is higher than the Nyquist limit, the signal begins to fold over on itself, or *alias,* resulting in a signal that is too distorted to be measured (Fig. 10-5). This technicality imposes limits on the maximum velocity of blood-flow that can be measured using pulsed-wave Doppler technology.

Continuous-Wave Mode

Continuous-wave Doppler technology employs two transducers, one for transmission and one for reception of the ultrasound signal. This dual system allows a continuous measurement of all the individual blood-flow velocities along the ultrasound beam but precludes gating based on depth; that is, it has no depth or range resolution. Continuous-wave Doppler can measure blood-flow velocities higher than pulsed-wave Doppler without aliasing (see Fig. 10-5) and is used primarily to determine the pressure gradient across a valve orifice. Continuous-wave Doppler does not allow a precise determination of velocity at a particular site within the heart.

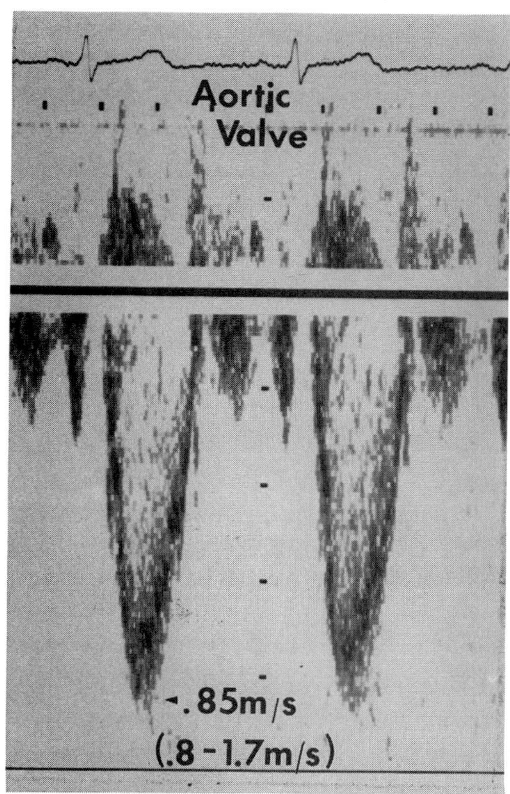

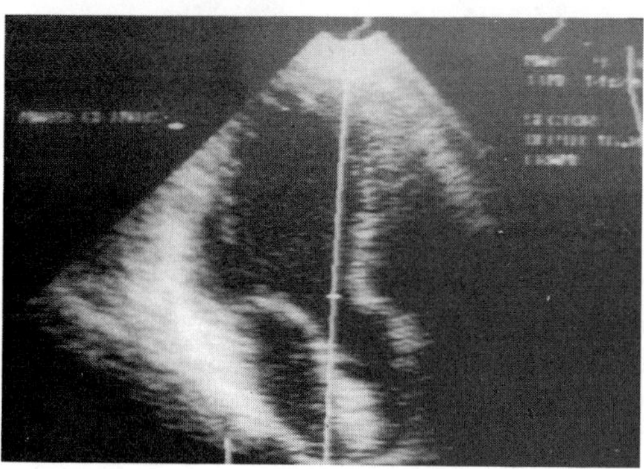

FIGURE 10-4. *Top,* The Doppler velocity curve derived from placement of a pulsed-wave sample volume at the level of the aortic valve. *Bottom,* The still frame, two-dimensional echocardiographic image demonstrates the location of the sample volume placement. *(Nishimura RA, Callahan MJ, Warnes CA: Echocardiography. In Giuliani ER, Fuster V, Gersh BJ, McGoon DC, McGoon MD (eds): Cardiology: Fundamentals and Practice, 2nd ed. Chicago, Year Book Medical Publishers [in press], by permission of Mayo Foundation)*

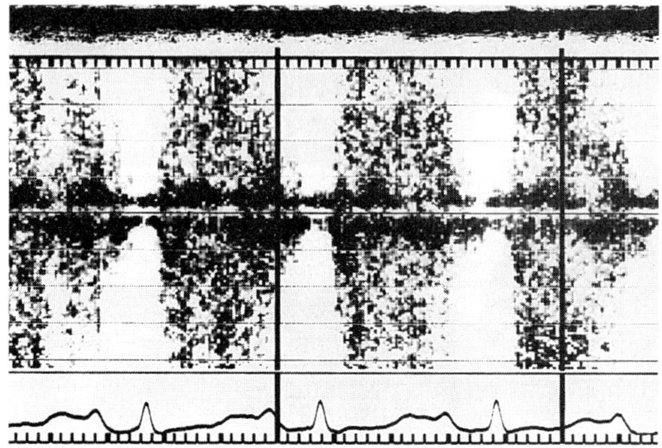

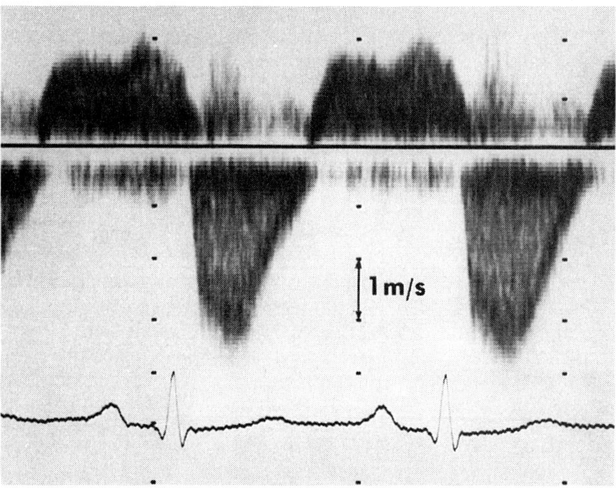

FIGURE 10-5. *Top,* The Doppler velocity curve of tricuspid regurgitation obtained by pulsed-wave Doppler. The velocity is higher than the pulse-repetition frequency. Thus aliasing occurs so that the peak velocity cannot be obtained. ***Bottom,*** A tricuspid regurgitation signal obtained by continuous-wave Doppler echocardiography. The peak velocity is clearly delineated. *(Nishimura RA, Callahan MJ, Warnes CA: Echocardiography. In Giuliani ER, Fuster V, Gersh BJ, McGoon DC, McGoon MD (eds): Cardiology: Fundamentals and Practice, 2nd ed. Chicago, Year Book Medical Publishers [in press], by permission of Mayo Foundation)*

Continuous-wave Doppler transducers are available as standalone systems or in combination with two-dimensional imaging capability (duplex system). The smaller, nonimaging transducer is frequently preferred over the larger duplex transducer because it allows imaging from more sites than does the larger probe.

APPLICATIONS OF DOPPLER TECHNOLOGY

Volumetric Flow

Ultrasonic Doppler techniques measure blood-flow velocity, which can be used to calculate volumetric flow rate. A pulsed-wave sample volume may be placed at a valve orifice or within a great vessel to obtain a Doppler velocity curve. The area under this Doppler velocity curve is termed the *time velocity integral* (TVI) (Fig. 10-6). The velocity is expressed in cm per second, and time is expressed in seconds. Therefore, the TVI represents the distance that blood moves in a given time period. The TVI multiplied by the cross-sectional area of the orifice (A), in this case the mitral valve annulus orifice, is equivalent to the stroke volume (SV) as shown in Equation 10-3.[5,6]

$$\mathrm{SV} = \mathrm{TVI} \cdot A \qquad (10\text{-}3)$$

In clinical circumstances, the area of an orifice is derived from a diameter measured from two-dimensional echocardiography. This calculation assumes a circular-shaped orifice with an area π d/2, where d equals the diameter of the orifice.

Calculation of volumetric flow by Doppler echocardiography makes the following assumptions: 1) blood flow through the heart valves or great vessels follows the principles of laminar flow through a rigid tube; 2) the orifice has a circular shape, which does not change throughout the cardiac cycle;[7,8] 3) the velocity profile through the orifice is flat and uniform;[9] and 4) the Doppler beam is parallel to the blood-flow vector. Despite these assumptions, numerous correlative studies have validated this technique for measurement of cardiac output.[10–16] With the use of precordial Doppler echocardiography, the best validation occurs when blood flow is measured at the level of the aortic valve annulus,[5] with satisfactory measurements being obtained in the left ventricular outflow tract,[11] ascending aorta,[12] descending aorta,[13,14] mitral valve,[15] pulmonary artery,[13] and tricuspid valve.[16] The advantages and disadvantages of the various sampling sites are reviewed elsewhere.[5,6,17]

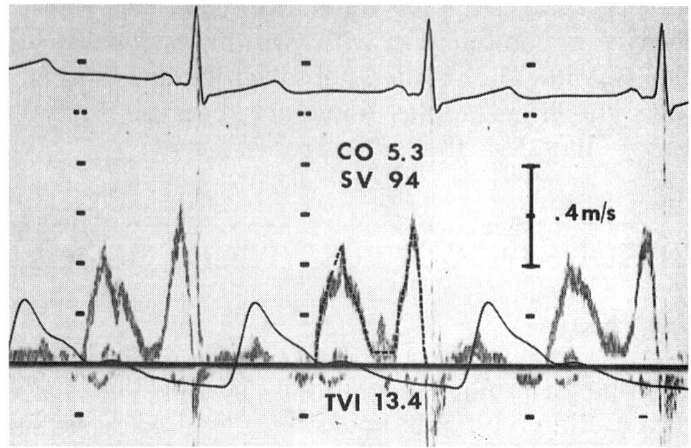

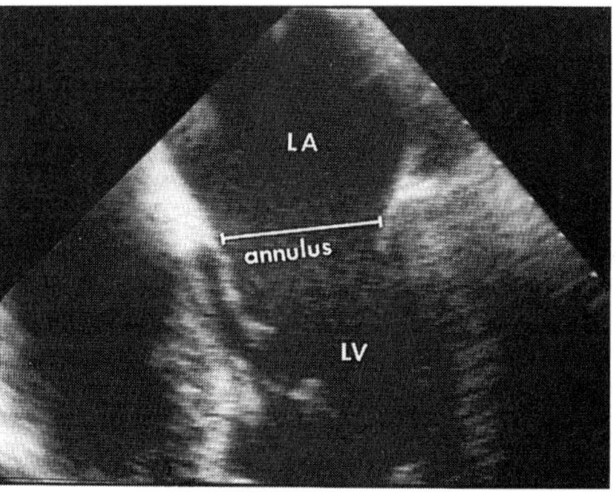

FIGURE 10-6. Calculation of cardiac output by Doppler echocardiography. *Top,* The mitral valve velocity curve obtained by a pulsed-wave sample volume placed at the level of the mitral valve annulus by transesophageal echocardiography. The dotted lines indicate the area underneath the curve, or the time-velocity integral (TVI). *Bottom,* Two-dimensional still frame transesophageal echocardiographic image demonstrates measurement of mitral valve annulus dimension. *Opposite,* Two-dimensional still frame transesophageal echocardiographic image demonstrates placement of the sample volume at the level of the mitral valve *(mv)* annulus. *LV,* left ventricle; *LA,* left atrium; *RV,* right ventricle; *CO,* cardiac output; *SV,* stroke volume. (continued)

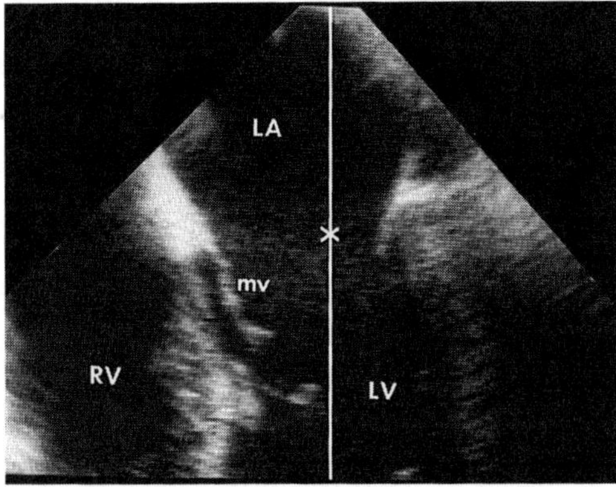

FIGURE 10-6 *(continued)*

the pulmonary artery can be imaged from the transesophageal position tages and disadvantages of the various sampling sites are reviewed elsewhere.[5,6,17]

In the operating room, transesophageal echocardiography (TEE) is superior to the precordial approach because it does not encroach on the surgical field and can be used continuously with minimal transducer manipulation. The initial experience used the descending thoracic aorta as the sampling site.[18–21] Limiting this technique is the need for preoperative calibration with a precordial Doppler cardiac output measurement because descending aortic blood-flow excludes approximately 40% of the cardiac output going to the arch vessels.[19] It is unlikely that the distribution of blood flow between arch vessels and the descending aorta remains constant over time, especially after cardiopulmonary bypass.[18] Thus, the usefulness of transesophageal measurements of blood flow in the descending aorta is limited.

The left ventricular outflow tract and ascending aorta cannot be used for cardiac output determination from the transesophageal position because it is difficult to line up the ultrasound beam parallel to the vector of blood flow. These limitations may be overcome with the development of the multiplanar transducers. The use of transmitral velocity measurements to determine cardiac output is an attractive alternative because of the close proximity of the mitral valve to the ultrasound transducer as well as the nearly parallel relationship between the direction of blood flow through the mitral valve annulus and the direction of the TEE Doppler beam (see Fig. 10-6). Initial studies that used this technique have demonstrated a fair correlation between Doppler cardiac output and thermodilution cardiac output.[22,23,23a] When

(70% of cases), cardiac output measurement that uses this site may be a more accurate way to determine cardiac output than the mitral valve method.[23]

Measurement of Pressure Gradient

The capability of measuring a pressure gradient across a valve is, in large part, responsible for the widespread use of Doppler ultrasound in cardiology. Measurement of the pressure gradient across an orifice is based on the Bernoulli equation, which describes the drop in pressure across an area of stenosis in terms of three component forces that contribute to the pressure drop (ΔP).[5] The equation can be summarized as shown in Equation 10-4.

$$\Delta P = P\text{ (convective acceleration)} + P\text{ (flow acceleration)} + P\text{ (viscous friction)} \qquad (10\text{-}4)$$

Convective acceleration occurs because of a change in the cross-sectional area of flow. The pressure drop due to convective acceleration may be thought of as the energy required to overcome the obstruction. The flow acceleration component of pressure causes a phase delay between the pressure drop and velocity curves and for clinical purposes is inconsequential.[25] If the orifice diameter is greater than 0.35 cm, then inertial forces (viscous friction component) are also negligible.[26–28] Thus, this equation can be simplified as shown in Equation 10-5,

$$\Delta P = P\text{ (convective acceleration)} \qquad (10\text{-}5)$$
$$P_1 - P_2 = \tfrac{1}{2} \cdot p \cdot (V_2^2 - V_1^2)$$

where $P_1 - P_2$ equals pressure drop across a stenotic area; p equals density of blood; V_1 equals velocity of blood before the stenosis; and V_2 equals velocity of blood after the stenosis. Because $V_1^2 \ll V_2^2$ it can be neglected, and because $\tfrac{1}{2} \cdot p = 4$, this equation can be simplified to Equation 10-6.

$$P_1 - P_2 = 4\ V_2^2 \qquad (10\text{-}6)$$

This modified form of the Bernoulli equation was first described by Holen and Hatle,[25–28] and its validity is supported by many additional studies.[29–33] The clinical utility of this equation is that it converts a blood-flow velocity ($\text{m}\cdot\text{s}^{-1}$) to a pressure gradient (mm Hg) across an orifice (Fig. 10-7).

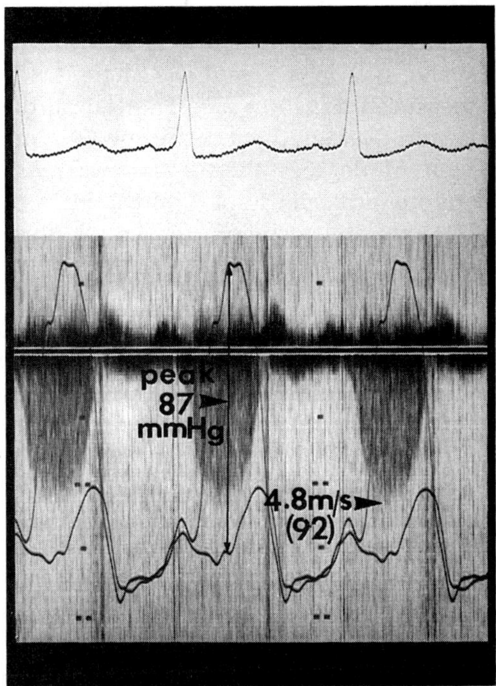

FIGURE 10-7. **A simultaneous mitral regurgitation velocity jet superimposed on the left ventricular and left atrial pressures. The gradient derived from the modified Bernoulli equation from the peak velocity of mitral regurgitation (92 mm Hg) corresponds to the peak gradient between the left ventricle and left atrium during systole (87 mm Hg).** *(Modified from Nishimura RA, Tajik AJ: Determination of left-sided pressure gradients by utilizing Doppler aortic and mitral regurgitant signals: Validation by simultaneous dual catheter and Doppler studies. J Am Coll Cardiol 11:317, 1988)*

Because of the exponential relationship between pressure drop and the velocity as described in the modified Bernoulli equation, the incident angle between the ultrasound beam and the blood-flow velocity vector (angle θ) must be as small as possible, particularly when estimating gradients across valve stenosis. Figure 10-3 and Table 10-1 demonstrate the relationship between velocity, pressure, and the angle θ. Using the example previously described, if the true peak velocity across a stenotic valve is 4 $m \cdot s^{-1}$, and the angle θ is 50 degrees, the peak velocity is measured as 2.6 $m \cdot s^{-1}$. Translating these data into a pressure drop, the true peak gradient would be 64 mm Hg; but, if the incident angle θ were 50 degrees, the measurement would be only 26 mm Hg. It is, therefore, critically important that every effort be made to obtain the true maximum velocity of a jet across a stenosis; any errors made because of a miscalculation of the velocity are exaggerated in the calculation of a pressure gradient.

It is usually not feasible to use TEE to assess high-pressure gradients intraoperatively because transesophageal ultrasound equipment has been limited mostly to pulsed-wave Doppler technology. As discussed previously, frequency aliasing occurs when high-velocity jets are analyzed with pulsed-wave Doppler, as seen with aortic stenosis, mitral regurgitation, and tricuspid regurgitation. The development of continuous-wave Doppler TEE probes with multiplane imaging capability should enable pressure gradient determinations from these high-velocity jets to be made in the near future. In mitral and tricuspid stenosis, however, the velocity may be low enough to allow measurement of the pressure gradients with pulsed-wave Doppler. This measurement results in accurate assessment of peak and mean gradients (Fig. 10-8).

Determination of Mitral Valve Area

The mitral valve gradients in mitral stenosis depend on the heart rate and cardiac output, as well as the degree of obstruction. Therefore, it is advantageous to be able to determine a valve area as a measure of severity. The effective mitral valve area can be determined with reasonable accuracy by using the slow rate of decline in the transmitral pressure gradient.[34] The rate of decline of the pressure gradient, a quadratic function of velocity, can be expressed by the time needed for the initial diastolic gradient to decline by 50% (pressure half-time [$t_{1/2}$]) (Fig. 10-9), as shown in Equation 10-7 (the Holen-Hatle modification of Bernoulli equation),

$$Pmax = 4\ Vmax^2 \qquad (10\text{-}7)$$

where *P*max equals maximum pressure gradient, and *V*max equals peak velocity of the transmitral diastolic flow. The $t_{1/2}$ is the time taken for

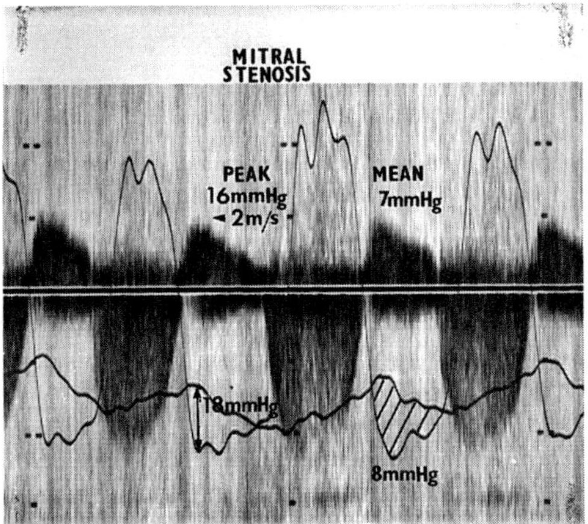

FIGURE 10-8. Simultaneous pressures and Doppler velocities from a patient with mitral stenosis. The pressures are from the left ventricle and pulmonary capillary wedge position. The Doppler velocity curve is typical of mitral stenosis with a high initial E velocity and a prolongation of the diastolic half-time. Both the peak pressure and the mean pressure gradients obtained from the Doppler velocity curves using the modified Bernoulli equation correspond to the simultaneous pressure gradients derived from cardiac catheterization. *(Brandenburg RO, Giuliani ER, Nishimura RA, McGood DC: Acquired valvular heart disease. In Giuliani ER, Fuster V, Gersh BJ, McGoon DC, McGoon MD (eds): Cardiology: Fundamentals and Practice, 2nd ed. Chicago, Year Book Medical Publishers [in press], by permission of Mayo Foundation)*

the pressure gradient to decrease to half Pmax, termed $Pt_{1/2}$ (Equation 10-8),

$$\tfrac{1}{2} \cdot P\text{max} = Pt_{1/2} = {V_{t_{1/2}}}^2 = \tfrac{1}{2} \cdot 4\ V\text{max}^2 \qquad (10\text{-}8)$$

where $V_{t_{1/2}}$ equals velocity of transmitral blood flow when the pressure gradient is ½ Pmax. The right side of this equation can be rearranged as in Equation 10-9.

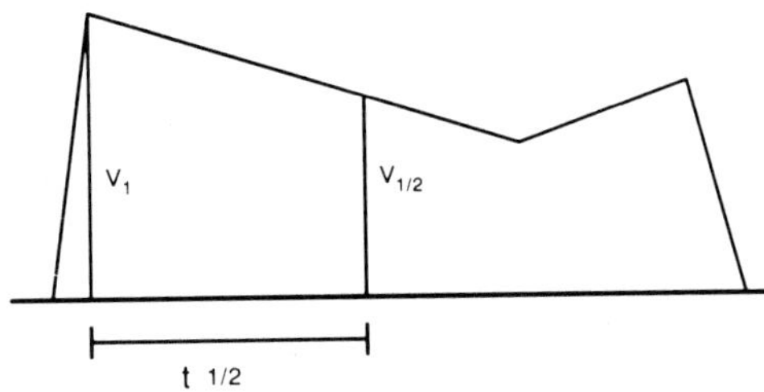

FIGURE 10-9. Schematic diagram of Doppler velocity curve in mitral stenosis illustrating the method for calculation of diastolic half time t½). V_1, maximum velocity in early diastole; $V_{1/2}$, velocity at which pressure gradient dropped by 50%.

$$V_{t_{1/2}} = \frac{V\text{max}}{\sqrt{2}} = \frac{V\text{max}}{1.4} \tag{10-9}$$

Thus, the velocity equivalent of half the maximum pressure gradient is obtained by dividing Vmax by 1.4. Once this value has been calculated, the point at which the mitral velocity decreases to this value is located. The time (millisecond) between Vmax and $V_{t_{1/2}}$ is the pressure half-time ($t_{1/2}$). The normal $t_{1/2}$ is 20 to 60 milliseconds. In mitral stenosis, it may range from 100 to 400 milliseconds, depending on the severity of the stenosis. The $t_{1/2}$ is inversely proportional to the mitral valve area, which is approximately 1 cm^2 at a $t_{1/2}$ of 220 milliseconds. Thus, if 220 is divided by the $t_{1/2}$, the mitral valve area can be calculated (Equation 10-10).[35]

$$\text{mitral valve area } (cm^2) = 220/t_{1/2} \tag{10-10}$$

The $t_{1/2}$ is inaccurate in patients with atrial tachycardia, prolonged PR interval, or coexistent severe aortic insufficiency. It is not influenced, however, by mitral regurgitation or varying RR intervals.[35]

Evaluation of Diastolic Function by Doppler Echocardiography

Abnormalities of diastolic function of the left ventricle may be an important cause of clinical symptomatology. In many conditions, diastolic dysfunction precedes the onset of abnormalities of systole. Dyspneic symptoms, for example, in patients with congestive heart failure, often are not attributable to diminished systolic performance but are probably due to diastolic abnormalities.[36,37] Diastolic filling of the heart is a complex sequence of multiple interrelated events, and it has been difficult in the past to measure parameters of diastolic function.

It is felt that Doppler interrogation of mitral valve velocities may provide an overall assessment of filling of the left ventricle. The transmitral velocity curve has two peaks, an early peak associated with rapid filling of the left ventricle, often termed the *E* velocity, and a late lower peak associated with atrial contraction, often termed the *A* velocity. After the E velocity, a linear decrease in velocity occurs. This rate of velocity fall can be measured by a deceleration time, which is the time from the mitral E velocity to the intersection of an extrapolation of this decline in velocity to the baseline (Fig. 10-10).

The position of the pulsed-wave Doppler sample volume influences the amplitude of the transmitral velocity curves. As the sample volume is moved from the left atrium to the mitral annulus toward the tips of the mitral valve leaflets, the peak velocities are increased (Fig. 10-11). Transmitral velocities are best recorded at the annulus for cardiac output measurements and at the tips of the mitral valve leaflets for assessment of diastolic function.

The transmitral velocity can be looked at as a function of the instantaneous pressure gradient between the left atrium and the left ventricle (Fig. 10-12).[38] Changes in the relationship between the left atrial and left ventricular pressures influence the profile of the transmitral velocities.[38–40] If left ventricular relaxation is prolonged, the initial gradient between the atrium and the ventricle is reduced, with a slower rate of fall of this gradient during mid-diastole. With less filling in early diastole, a greater proportion of filling in late diastole at atrial contraction occurs.[38] Thus, the E velocity is smaller, the rate of decline of the E velocity (deceleration time) is decreased, and the A velocity is increased. An abnormal relaxation pattern is characterized by the presence of low E velocity, low E-A ratio, and a prolongation of the deceleration time (Fig. 10-13).[38] An abnormal relaxation pattern has been noted in patients with hypertrophic cardiomyopathy, hypertension, and coronary artery disease.[41–44]

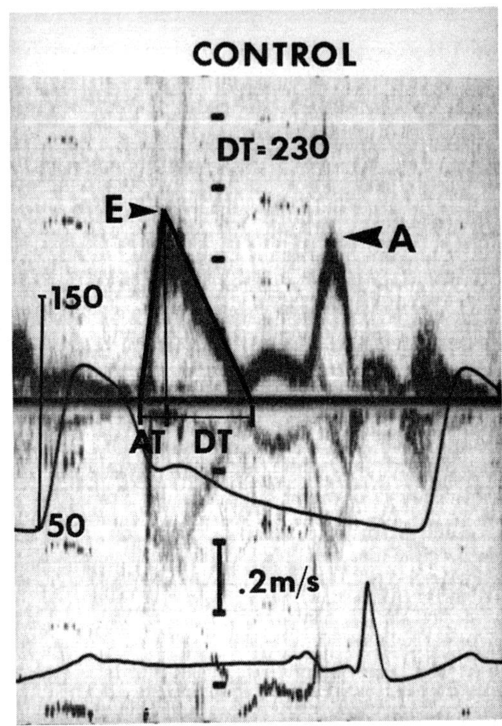

FIGURE 10-10. The mitral flow velocity curve in a normal patient, illustrating measurement of *E* velocity, *A* velocity, and deceleration time *(DT)*. The simultaneous radial artery pressure is shown with a calibration scale of 50 to 150 mm Hg. *(Nishimura RA, Abel MD, Housmans PR, Warnes CA: Mitral flow velocity curves as a function of different loading conditions: Evaluation by intraoperative transesophageal Doppler echocardiography. J Am Society of Echocardiography 2:79, 1989, by permission of the American Society of Echocardiography)*

A decrease in left ventricular compliance, on the other hand, results in a rapid rise in the left ventricular diastolic pressure early in diastole. The higher initial left atrial pressure causes a high initial velocity, or E wave. A short deceleration time is due to the rapid rise in left ventricular pressure, which rapidly approximates or becomes higher than left atrial pressure.[38] In patients with restrictive,[45] dilated, hypertrophic, or ischemic cardiomyopathy, a particular pattern of transmitral

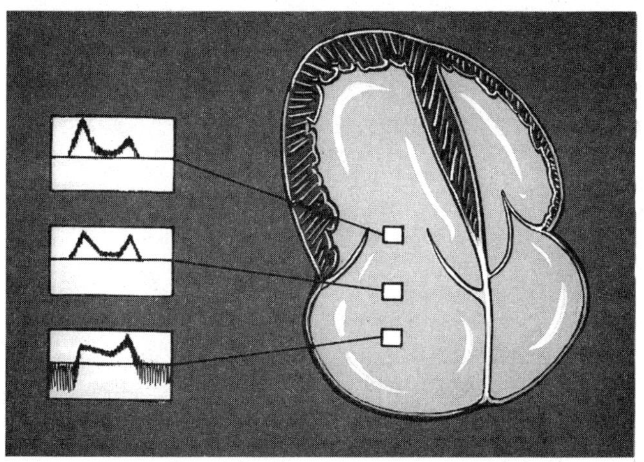

FIGURE 10-11. The mitral flow velocity curves change in their configuration as the sample volume is placed into the left ventricle at the mitral valve leaflet tips, the mitral valve annulus, and into the left atrium.

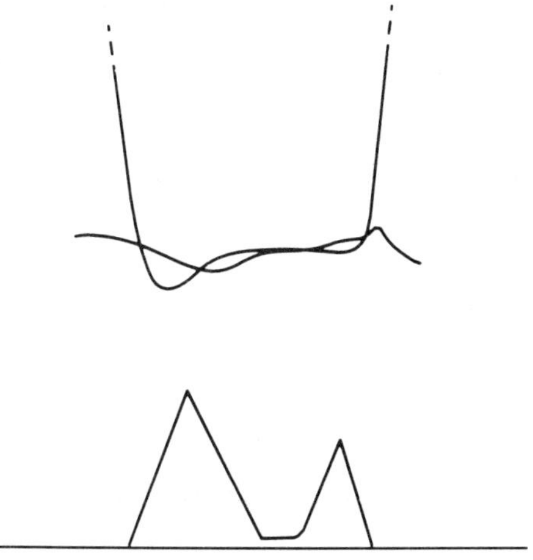

FIGURE 10-12. Schematic diagram of the mitral valve flow velocity curve *(bottom)* and simultaneous left ventricular and left atrial pressures *(top)*. *(Nishimura RA, Abel MD, Hatle LK, Tajik AJ: Assessment of diastolic function of the heart: Background and current applications of Doppler echocardiography. Part II. Clinical studies. Mayo Clin Proc 64:181, 1989)*

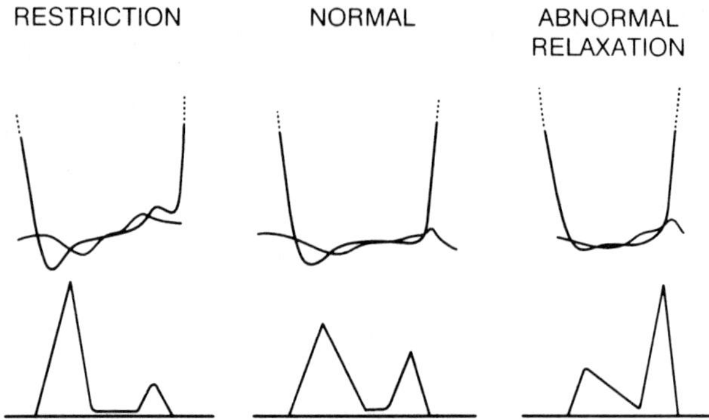

FIGURE 10-13. Schematic diagram of the three types of mitral flow velocity curves and the corresponding left ventricular–left atrial pressures that are seen in clinical practice. *(Modified from Nishimura RA, Abel MD, Hatle LK, Tajik AJ: Assessment of diastolic function of the heart: Background and current application of Doppler echocardiography. Part II. Clinical studies. Mayo Clin Proc 64:181, 1989)*

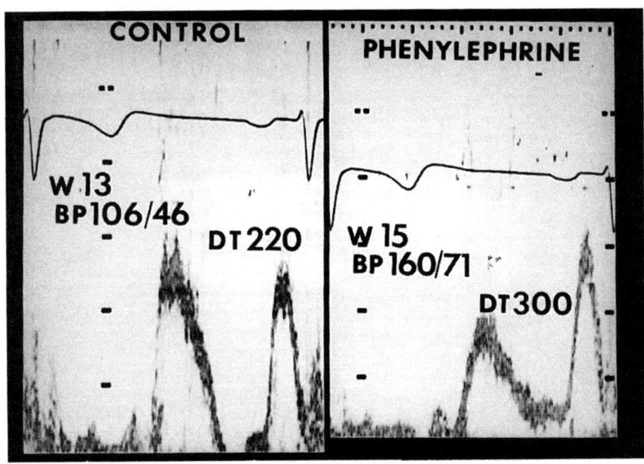

FIGURE 10-14. Demonstration of the change in the mitral flow velocity curve in the control state and after an increase in blood pressure by phenylephrine. A decrease in the initial velocity, a prolongation of deceleration time *(DT)*, and a decrease in E-A ratio occur. *W*, pulmonary capillary wedge pressure; *BP*, blood pressure. *(Nishimura RA, Abel MD, Hatle LK, Tajik AJ: Relationship of pulmonary vein to mitral flow velocities by transesophageal Doppler echocardiography: Effect of different loading conditions. Circulation 81:1488, 1990, by permission of Mayo Foundation)*

velocity termed *restriction to filling* frequently is seen. This pattern is characterized by a high E velocity, a short deceleration time, and a relatively small A velocity, and, thus, a high E-A ratio (see Fig. 10-13).[38] The effect of atrial contraction depends on left ventricular diastolic pressure before atrial contraction.[46–48] Diastolic mitral regurgitation may also occur.[45]

Factors other than abnormalities of left ventricular diastolic function influence the pattern of transmitral velocities. These factors include preload and afterload[38,40,49,50] and heart rate.[51,52] Figure 10-13 demonstrates how the transmitral velocity profile may be altered in the same patient by simply altering loading conditions.[38] Increases in afterload produce a pattern similar to a relaxation abnormality (Fig. 10-14), while increases in preload produce a velocity curve that is quite similar to that seen in patients with a restriction to filling (Fig. 10-15). An abnormal relaxation pattern can be pseudonormalized by fluid administration with concomitant elevation of the left atrial pressure.

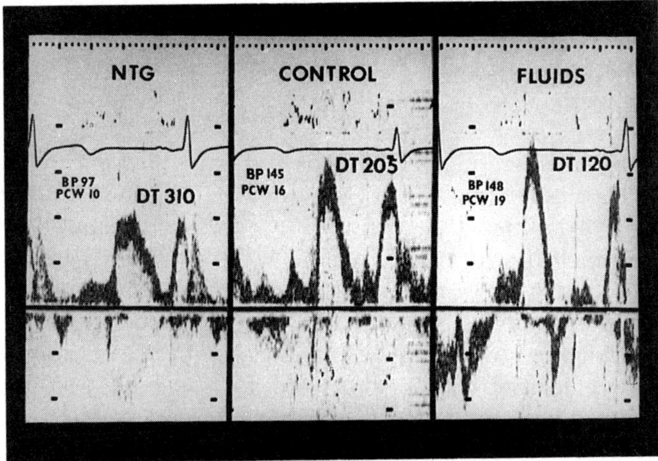

FIGURE 10-15. The mitral flow velocity curves demonstrate the changes that occur with changes in filling pressures. ***Left,*** Low filling pressure with intravenous nitroglycerin (NTG). ***Center,*** Control state. ***Right,*** High filling pressures from infusion of fluids. ***BP,*** blood pressure; ***PCW,*** pulmonary capillary wedge pressure; ***DT,*** deceleration time. *(Nishimura RA, Abel MD, Housmans PR, Warnes CA: Mitral flow velocity curves as a function of different loading conditions: evaluation by intraoperative transesophageal Doppler echocardiography. J Am Society of Echocardiography 2:79, 1989, by permission of the American Society of Echocardiography)*

The significant influence that loading conditions and heart rate have on transmitral velocity leads to the concept that specific Doppler patterns exist within particular hemodynamic classes of patients rather than within specific disease groups.[53–55] The influence of changes in loading conditions on transmitral velocity may allow anesthesiologists to determine noninvasively the change in loading conditions of the left ventricle.

Pulmonary Vein-Flow Velocities

Blood flow into the left atrium has a characteristic profile that can be evaluated by a pulsed-wave sample volume placed in the pulmonary vein (Fig. 10-16).[56–58] Flow into the left atrium occurs with its relaxation and in association with the descent of the atrioventricular valves during ventricular systole. This is followed by a diastolic inflow, which is influenced by the same parameters that determine the mitral valve E and deceleration time. Atrial contraction produces flow reversal from the left atrium into the pulmonary vein, the A velocity. With TEE, it has become feasible to visualize the pulmonary veins routinely, an act that is often difficult to achieve with the transthoracic approach.[59] Commonly, the left upper lobe pulmonary vein can be imaged from the transesophageal position, and the pulsed-wave Doppler ultrasound beam can be aligned parallel to the direction of blood flow. Several studies have examined the relationship of the pulmonary vein-flow velocity parameters with hemodynamic indices.[60,61] The cardiac output and pulmonary artery wedge pressure correlate with the systolic and atrial components of the pulmonary vein flow velocity respectively.[60] The left atrial pressure inversely correlates with the pulmonary vein systolic-flow velocity fraction of forward flow.[61]

Pulmonary vein-flow velocities have also been used in an effort to estimate the severity of mitral regurgitation. The magnitude of flow reversal during ventricular systole has been suggested as a method of determining severity of mitral regurgitation.[62] However, this parameter may be more dependent on the direction of the regurgitant jet rather than the severity of regurgitation.

Additional studies need to be done to evaluate further the usefulness of pulsed-wave Doppler parameters of diastolic function. It is hoped that an estimate of left ventricular filling pressure will be obtainable based on an analysis of the transmitral and pulmonary vein-flow velocity curves obtained with transesophageal pulsed-wave Doppler echocardiography.

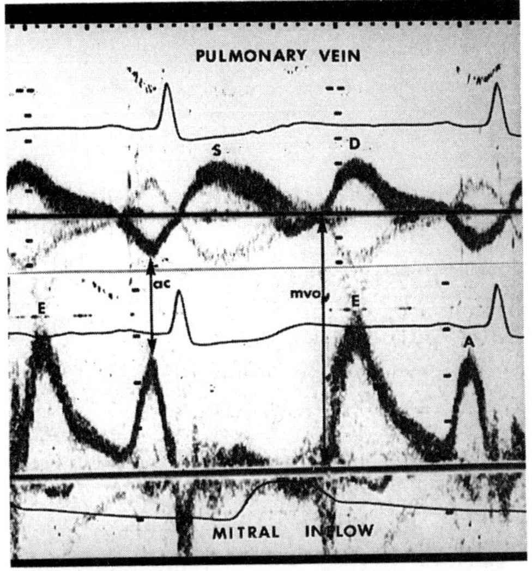

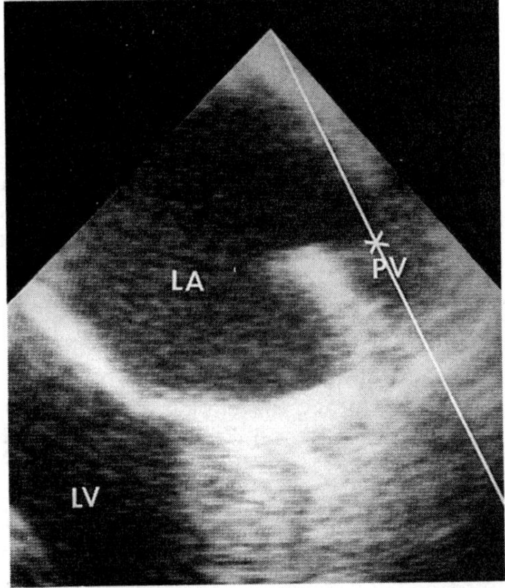

FIGURE 10-16. *Top,* The velocity curve obtained from placement of the sample volume in the pulmonary vein by transesophageal echocardiography. The relationship to the mitral-flow velocity is shown. ***Bottom,*** Still frame transesophageal echocardiographic picture demonstrates placement of the sample volume in the pulmonary vein (PV). ***LA,*** left atrium; ***LV,*** left ventricle; ***AC,*** atrial contraction. *(Top: Modified from Nishimura RA, Abel MD, Hatle LK, Tajik AJ: Relation of pulmonary vein to mitral flow velocities by transesophageal Doppler echocardiography: Effect of different loading conditions. Circulation 81:1488, 1990, by permission of Mayo Foundation)*

CONCLUSION

The use of Doppler echocardiography in association with TEE has significantly enhanced both the diagnostic and monitoring capabilities of this new form of imaging. Doppler echocardiography can be used to estimate cardiac output, pressure gradients across valve orifices, valve area, and, potentially, left ventricular filling pressures.

References

1. Gillispie CC: Dictionary of Scientific Biography, Vol IV, pp. 167–168. New York, Charles Scribner's Sons, 1971
2. Hatle L, Angelsen B: Doppler Ultrasound in Cardiology, 2nd edition, pp. 1–7. Philadelphia, Lea & Febiger, 1985
3. Lorch G, Rubenstein S, Baker D, Dooley T, Dodge H: Doppler echocardiography: Use of a graphical display system. Circulation 56:576, 1977
4. Nishimura RA, Miller FA, Callahan MJ et al: Doppler echocardiography: Theory, instrumentation, technique and application. Mayo Clin Proc 60:320, 1985
5. Zoghbi WA, Quinones MA: Determination of cardiac output by Doppler echocardiography: A critical appraisal. Herz 11:258, 1986
6. Sahn DJ, Valdes Cruz LM: Ultrasound Doppler methods for calculating cardiac volume flows, cardiac output, and cardiac shunts. Cardiovasc Clin 17:19, 1986
7. Ormiston JA, Shah PM, Tei C, Wong M: Size and motion of the mitral valve annulus in man. Part I. A two-dimensional echocardiographic method and findings in normal subjects. Circulation 64:113, 1981
8. Tsakiris AG, von Bernuth G, Rastelli GC, Bourgeois MJ, Titus JL, Wood EH: Size and motion of the mitral valve annulus in anesthetized intact dogs. J Appl Physiol 30:611, 1971
9. Samstad SO, Torp H, Linker DT et al: Cross-sectional instantaneous flow velocity profiles by two-dimensional Doppler ultrasound applied to early mitral flow in normals (abstr). Circulation 78 (suppl):113, 1988
10. Looyenga DS, Liebson PR, Bone RC, Balk RA, Messer JV: Determination of cardiac output in critically ill patients by dual beam Doppler echocardiography. J Am Coll Cardiol 13:340, 1989
11. Lewis JF, Kuo LC, Nelson JG, Limacher MC, Quinones MA: Pulsed Doppler echocardiographic determination of stroke volume and cardiac output: Clinical validation of two new methods using the apical window. Circulation 70:425, 1984
12. Dittmann H, Voelker W, Karsch K-R, Seipel L: Influence of sampling site and flow area on cardiac output measurements by Doppler echocardiography. J Am Coll Cardiol 10:818, 1987
13. Labovitz AJ, Buckingham TA, Habermehl K, Nelson J, Kennedy HL, Williams GA: The effects of sampling site on the two-dimensional echo-Doppler determination of cardiac output. Am Heart J 109:327, 1985
14. Smith HJ, Grottum P, Simonsen S: Doppler flowmetry in the lower tho-

racic aorta: An indirect estimation of cardiac output. Acta Radiol [suppl] (Stockh) 26:257, 1985

15. Hoit BD, Rashwan M, Watt C, Sahn DJ, Bhargava V: Calculating cardiac output from transmitral volume flow using Doppler and M-mode echocardiography. Am J Cardiol 62:131, 1988
16. Meijboom EJ, Horowitz S, Valdes-Cruz LM, Sahn DJ, Larson DF, Oliveira Lima C: A Doppler echocardiographic method for calculating volume flow across the tricuspid valve: Correlative laboratory and clinical studies. Circulation 71:551, 1985
17. Sahn DJ: Determination of cardiac output by echocardiographic Doppler methods: Relative accuracy of various sites for measurement. J Am Coll Cardiol 6:663, 1985
18. Mark JB, Steinbrook RA, Gugino LD et al: Continuous noninvasive monitoring of cardiac output with esophageal Doppler ultrasound during cardiac surgery. Anesth Analg 65:1013, 1986
19. Freund PR: Transesophageal Doppler scanning versus thermodilution during general anesthesia: An initial comparison of cardiac output techniques. Am J Surg 153:490, 1987
20. Hillel Z, Thys D, Keene D, Snook D, Lasker S: A method to improve the accuracy of esophageal Doppler cardiac output determinations (abstr). Anesthesiology 71:A386, 1989
21. Perrino AC, Fleming J, LaMantia KR: Advances in Doppler technology improve cardiac output monitoring (abstr). Anesthesiology 71:A349, 1989
22. LaMantia K, Harris S, Mortimore K, Davis E, Barash PG: Transesophageal pulse-wave Doppler assessment of cardiac output (abstr). Anesthesiology 69:A1, 1988
23. Muhiudeen IA, Kuecherer HF, Lee E, Cahalan MK, Schiller NB: Transesophageal Doppler echocardiography for monitoring cardiac output (abstr). Anesthesiology 71:A389, 1989

23a. Abel MD, Nishimura RA, Ereth MA, Ilstrup D: Determination of cardiac output intraoperatively by transesophageal Doppler echocardiography. Anesthesiology (submitted for publication)

24. Hatle L, Angelsen B: Doppler Ultrasound in Cardiology, 2nd edition, pp. 8–31. Philadelphia, Lea & Febiger, 1985
25. Holen J, Aaslid R, Landmark K, Simonsen S, Ostrem T: Determination of effective orifice area in mitral stenosis from non-invasive ultrasound Doppler data and mitral flow rate. Acta Med Scand 201:83, 1977
26. Holen J, Aaslid R, Landmark K, Simonsen S: Determination of pressure gradient in mitral stenosis with a non-invasive ultrasound Doppler technique. Acta Med Scand 199:455, 1976
27. Hatle L, Brubakk AO, Tromsdal A, Angelsen B: Noninvasive assessment of pressure drop in mitral stenosis by Doppler ultrasound. Br Heart J 40:131, 1978
28. Hatle L, Angelsen BA, Tromsdal A: Non-invasive assessment of aortic stenosis by Doppler ultrasound. Br Heart J 43:284, 1980
29. Callahan MJ, Tajik AJ, Su-Fan Q, Bove AA: Continuous wave Doppler-catheterization correlation of pressure gradients in experimental aortic stenosis (abstr). Circulation 70 (suppl):114, 1984
30. Stamm BR, Martin RP: Quantification of pressure gradients across stenotic valves by Doppler ultrasound. J Am Coll Cardiol 2:707, 1984

31. Berger M, Berdoff RL, Gallerstein PE, Goldberg E: Evaluation of aortic stenosis by continuous wave ultrasound. J Am Coll Cardiol 3:150, 1984
32. Lima CO, Sahn DJ, Valdes-Cruz LM et al: Prediction of the severity of left ventricular outflow tract obstruction by quantitative two-dimensional echocardiographic Doppler studies. Circulation 68:348, 1983
33. Nishimura RA, Tajik AJ: Determination of left-sided pressure gradients by utilizing Doppler aortic and mitral regurgitant signals: Validation by simultaneous dual catheter and Doppler studies. J Am Coll Cardiol 11:317, 1988
34. Libanoff AJ, Rodbard S: Atrioventricular pressure half-time: Measure of mitral valve orifice area. Circulation 38:144, 1968
35. Hatle L, Angelsen B, Tromsdal A: Noninvasive assessment of atrioventricular pressure half-time by Doppler ultrasound. Circulation 60:1096, 1979
36. Dodek A, Kassebaum DG, Bristow JD: Pulmonary edema in coronary artery disease without cardiomegaly: Paradox of the stiff heart. N Engl J Med 286:1347, 1972
37. Dougherty AH, Naccarelli GV, Gray EL, Hicks CH: Congestive heart failure with normal systolic function. Am J Cardiol 54:778, 1984
38. Nishimura RA, Abel MD, Hatle LK, Tajik AJ: Assessment of diastolic function of the heart: Background and current applications of Doppler echocardiography. Part II. Clinical studies. Mayo Clin Proc 64:181, 1989
39. Nishimura RA, Housmans PR, Hatle LK, Tajik AJ: Assessment of diastolic function of the heart: Background and current applications of Doppler echocardiography. Part I. Physiologic and pathophysiologic features. Mayo Clin Proc 64:71, 1989
40. Nishimura RA, Abel MD, Hatle LK, Holmes DR Jr, Housman PR, Ritman EL, Tajik AJ: Significance of Doppler indices of diastolic filling of the left ventricle: Comparison with invasive hemodynamics in a canine model (abstr). Am Heart J 118(6):1248, 1989
41. Kitabatake A, Inoue M, Asao M et al: Transmitral blood flow reflecting diastolic behavior of the left ventricle in health and disease: A study by pulsed Doppler technique. Jpn Circ J 46:92, 1982
42. Pearson AC, Labovitz AJ, Mrosek D, Williams GA, Kennedy HL: Assessment of diastolic function in normal and hypertrophied hearts: Comparison of Doppler echocardiography and M-mode echocardiography. Am Heart J 113:1417, 1987
43. Wind BE, Snider AR, Buda AJ, O'Neill WW, Topol EJ, Dilworth LR: Pulsed Doppler assessment of left ventricular diastolic filling in coronary artery disease before and immediately after coronary angioplasty. Am J Cardiol 59:1041, 1987
44. Bryg RJ, Pearson AC, Williams GA, Labovitz AJ: Left ventricular systolic and diastolic flow abnormalities determined by Doppler echocardiography in obstructive hypertrophic cardiomyopathy. Am J Cardiol 59:925, 1987
45. Appleton CP, Hatle LK, Popp RL: Demonstration of restrictive ventricular physiology by Doppler echocardiography. J Am Coll Cardiol 11:757, 1988
46. Greenberg B, Chatterjee K, Parmley WM, Werner JA, Holly AN: The influence of left ventricular filling pressure on atrial contribution to cardiac output. Am Heart J 98:742, 1979

47. Channer KS, Culling W, Wilde P, Jones JV: Estimation of left ventricular end-diastolic pressure by pulsed Doppler ultrasound. Lancet 1:1005, 1986
48. Bristow JD, Van Zee BE, Judkins MP: Systolic and diastolic abnormalities of the left ventricle in coronary artery disease: Studies in patients with little or no enlargement of ventricular volume. Circulation 42:219, 1970
49. Nishimura RA, Abel MD, Housmans PR, Warnes CA: Mitral flow velocity curves as a function of different loading conditions: Evaluation by intraoperative transesophageal Doppler echocardiography. Journal of the American Society of Echocardiography 2:79, 1989
50. Abel MD, Nishimura RA: Assessment of diastolic function by transesophageal pulsed Doppler echocardiography: Effect of different loading conditions on mitral inflow velocities during coronary bypass surgery. In Erbel R, Khandheria BK, Brennecke R, Meyer J, Seward JB, Tajik AJ (eds): Transesophageal Echocardiography: A New Window to the Heart, p. 282. Berlin, Springer-Verlag, 1989
51. Smith SA, Stoner JE, Russell AE, Sheppard JM, Aylward PE: Transmitral velocities measured by pulsed Doppler in healthy volunteers: Effects of acute changes in blood pressure and heart rate. Br Heart J 61:344, 1989
52. Gillam LD, Homma S, Novick S, Rediker DE, Eagle KA: The influence of heart rate on Doppler mitral inflow patterns (abstr). Circulation 76 (suppl):123, 1987
53. Choong CY, Herrmann HC, Weyman AE, Fifer MA: Preload dependence of Doppler-derived indexes of left ventricular diastolic function in humans. J Am Coll Cardiol 10:800, 1987
54. Appleton CP, Hatle LK, Popp RL: Relation of transmitral flow velocity patterns to left ventricular diastolic function: New insights from a combined hemodynamic and Doppler echocardiographic study. J Am Coll Cardiol 12:426, 1988
55. Choong CY, Abascal VM, Thomas JD, Guerrero JL, McGlew S, Weyman AE: Combined influence of ventricular loading and relaxation on the transmitral flow velocity profile in dogs measured by Doppler echocardiography. Circulation 78:672, 1988
56. Keren G, Sherez J, Megidish R, Levitt B, Laniado S: Pulmonary venous flow pattern—its relationship to cardiac dynamics: A pulsed Doppler echocardiographic study. Circulation 71:1105, 1985
57. Keren G, Bier A, Sherez J, Miura D, Keefe D, LeJemtel T: Atrial contraction is an important determinant of pulmonary venous flow. J Am Coll Cardiol 7:693, 1986
58. Keren G, Sonnenblick EH, LeJemtel TH: Mitral annulus motion: Relaxation to pulmonary venous and transmitral flows in normal subjects and in patients with dilated cardiomyopathy. Circulation 78:621, 1988
59. Seward JB, Khandheria BK, Oh JK et al: Transesophageal echocardiography: Technique, anatomic correlations, implementation, and clinical applications. Mayo Clin Proc 63:649, 1988
60. Nishimura RA, Abel MD, Hatle LK, Tajik AJ: Relation of pulmonary vein to mitral flow velocities by transesophageal Doppler echocardiography. Effect of different loading conditions. Circulation 81:1488, 1990
61. Kuecherer HF, Muhiudeen IA, Lee E, Cahalan MK, Schiller NB: Estimation of left atrial pressure by Doppler interrogation of phasic pulmonary

venous flow: An intraoperative transesophageal study (abstr). Circulation 80 (suppl):566, 1989

62. Klein AL, Obarski TP, Calafiore PC et al: Reversal of flow in pulmonary veins by transesophageal echocardiography predicts severity of mitral regurgitation. Presented at the International Symposium on Cardiovascular Ultrasound: Applications of New Technologies, Rochester, MN, September 17–20, 1989

Index

Page numbers followed by (*t*) indicate tables; page numbers followed by (*f*) indicate figures.

ISBN 0-397-51128-0